CW00866300

Outside the Dissecting Room

Outside the Dissecting Room

DAVID SINCLAIR

Former Regius Professor of Anatomy, University of Aberdeen
and Emeritus Professor at the University of Western Australia

RADCLIFFE MEDICAL PRESS

OXFORD

© 1989 Radcliffe Medical Press Ltd
15 Kings Meadow, Ferry Hinksey Road, Oxford OX2 ODP

British Library Cataloguing in Publication Data
Sinclair, David

ISBN 1 870905 06 7

Printed and bound in Great Britain
Typeset by Advance Typesetting, Oxfordshire

Contents

Foreword

When the proofs of this book arrived from the publisher I was enjoying a particularly leisurely spell of retirement. The phone had not rung for at least an hour with some distress call from a beleagured organisation, flatteringly implying that its imminent collapse could be averted only by a transfusion of my supposedly magic formula for salvation. I had only one book and five promised articles to write, only nine typescripts of books and sundry other texts lay on my desk requiring, I had been assured, no more than my deathless comments to transform them into winners which no publisher or editor could possibly spurn; and the number of committees I was due to chair in the coming week was in single figures. Moreover I could look forward to tranquil nights broken only by the need to venture out in the small hours to water the drought-ravaged garden, cloaked in a darkness that minimised the risk of detection by the privatised water company's low-flying spotter plane. So before getting down to the article heaviest on my conscience, I picked up the proofs. Several hours passed in nostalgic enjoyment and the article was postponed yet again.

Many of these pieces by David Sinclair first appeared under the heading 'In England Now' in *The Lancet*. For many years after that column began in the journal, in the early days of the 1939–45 war, it virtually ran itself. Before long, material streamed in from far and near. The editorial task was simply to choose the best. So when readers said to the then Editor (as they often did) ''The first thing I read in your journal is 'In England Now' '' he was less gratified than they hoped he would be because it was not the part of the journal on which the greatest editorial creativity was lavished. Anyway, David Sinclair was the star of 'In England Now' in its heyday. When it somehow lost its vigour after twenty years or so it wasn't his fault. Much of its vitality lay in the multiplicity of contributors; and eventually they seemed to go elsewhere, perhaps to *World Medicine* and other new journals. For reasons I find it hard to identify now (perhaps it was the preoccupation of a small staff with a flood of papers and letters), *The Lancet* did little to counter this loss. When it came to make a deliberate effort to revive the column, ten years or so ago, I was fortunate to have the help of a few friends who enjoyed writing in this vein and wrote well, among them the irreplaceable David Sinclair. His life, professedly that of a humdrum academic, has apparently been studded with encounters and adventures from which he has extracted tales of hilarious misfortune; and he can expand little oddities into full-blown laughter. In providing a leavening of wit in an increasingly heavy dough of medical science, he has heartened many readers and at least one editor.

IAN MUNRO
Editor, *The Lancet*, 1976–88

Preface

Students of medicine and the medical sciences find their preclinical teachers mystifying, particularly those who have a
medical degree. They can see how it might happen that an
unambitious and not too bright chap could become trapped into
becoming a professor of medicine or surgery, but they cannot
imagine how anyone qualified in medicine and with an average
intelligence quotient could possibly contemplate embracing a
subject like anatomy as a career.

I hope that this book may serve to show them that preclinical
teachers, even of anatomy, are human beings after all, and
perhaps it may also entertain some of those who, as medical,
nursing or paramedical workers, may have strayed far from the
peaceful ambience of the lecture room and laboratory. Some
people outside the medical professions altogether may be
interested to find that contributing to the early stages of medical
education is not a task of unrelieved seriousness and high
purpose.

Most of the pieces are contributions made between 1948 and
1988 to the column 'In England Now' in the Lancet, and I am
grateful to the publishers for permission to reprint them. A few
have been expanded, and some hitherto unpublished material
has been included.

My working life has been divided between Britain and
Australia, and this accounts for the varying backgrounds of the
experiences I have recorded. Despite their varying attributions,
most of them are my own.

DAVID SINCLAIR
August, 1989

Departments and Denizens

The Grand Design

WE spoke the other day to a normally inoffensive and retiring chap who looks after one of the more arcane departments in the medical school. As befitted his lowly status, our colleague had been immured for many years in what is laughingly called temporary accommodation, and he was therefore delighted when without warning the planning of a new and more substantial building was authorised. He was graciously allowed to inspect the architect's plans, which naturally had discarded every one of the exceedingly well-considered requirements he had submitted. Having no previous experience of this law of nature, he became quite excited, and, insofar as his temperament allowed it, steam came out of his ears. He prepared some astringent comments for the relevant meeting of the buildings committee, to which he found that the architect had brought a scale model, painted in pastel shades and surrounded by improbable plastic trees.

The architect was tall and slender, and gave the impression that he would be happier among flying buttresses and clerestory windows; he directed his exposition entirely to the model and not to the plans. 'The building reads from the outside in terms of its function', said the architect. (Since function had been totally ignored, our colleague could make nothing of this.) 'It is not neutral in aesthetics', went on the architect, 'the building speaks'. (Our colleague's blood pressure rose still further, and he ground his teeth.) Swivelling deferentially round to the Vice-Chancellor, the architect continued: 'There is a great deal of tension in the design, which is given expression in the finishes and in the multitude of different elements'.

The buildings committee had clearly been through this sort of thing many times, but our colleague had not, and when his turn came to speak his emotions boiled over into an impassioned diatribe. He pointed out that he and his staff had to live inside, not outside, the building, that the internal arrangements were totally unsatisfactory, and that the most childish errors of design had been perpetrated. The architect flushed and bridled; some of our colleague's barbs had hit home. But eventually things were smoothed over, and revised interior plans were approved. Our colleague was even consulted about the internal colour scheme, and chose suitably innocuous floor coverings, curtains and wall paint; he was not asked to consider the service ducts and pipes for the architect said, *ex cathedra*, 'We must solve the colour problem test-wise.'

It was therefore with considerable satisfaction that our colleague˙ rashly departed on leave. On his return to take possession of his new domain, he found that in his absence the colour problem had been solved test-wise in a somewhat basic fashion. The giant inflow ducts of the air-conditioning system, which dominated the ceilings of every room, had been painted an electric scarlet. The companion outflow ducts immediately alongside were a vicious blue, and the exposed pipes of the plumbing a bilious yellow. The water pipes were bright green and the gas supply bright purple.

The screaming psychedelic sunbursts proved impossible to subdue, for all the money had been spent, so it appears that the Architect's Revenge will last for an indefinite period. Students with petit mal have been counselled to avoid the classroom, and our colleague has bought a pair of dark glasses.

St. Mildred's Revenge

WE have had the builders in for some time now, hammering and bumping away, and we are beginning to show signs of what our French visitor calls 'le Stress.' The first thing to go was our internal telephone. It began insidiously, by doing little sums to itself, so that when we dialled 518 we got 629. Inspired by our statistician, we started doing our own little sums before we dialled, and for a time we had it baffled. But now when we lift the receiver we find ourselves in an echoing cavern populated by rattles and howls. We can occasionally identify the voices of our colleagues across the gulf, but our efforts to place ourselves in communication with them are in vain. The other day the mad thought came to us that we would like to speak to Pharmacology, and we superimposed the appropriate number on the prevailing chaos. To our surprise there was immediate silence, and we could hear someone breathing heavily. 'Hello,' we said politely, 'is that Pharmacology?' 'Neither now nor at any time has it been Pharmacology,' said a voice unpleasantly close to our ear, 'this is the library basement. Why don't you get something *done* about your damned telephone?'

Nor is this all. Yesterday morning, just as we were passing the lecture-room, the rotary polisher broke away from the restraining hands of our industrious cleaner and made its way, lurching and growling, out of the lecture-room door to the hall, where it pinned the professor into one corner under the coat racks. Still kicking and buzzing spitefully, it was dragged off its prey by our resourceful secretary, and eventually silenced by cutting off the current, but not before a deep impression had been created.

Then there is the affair of the letter. We are used to receiving letters from overseas addressed to us at London, Oxford, or even London, Germany (we do not live in London), but until last week we had never had a letter addressed to us with the simple word 'deceased' following our medical qualifications. It gave us quite a turn.

At last, however, we have an explanation of these occurrences. The builders have unearthed, from a cupboard scheduled for demolition, a small cardboard box labelled 'Medieval teeth (St. Mildred's).' It is clear that St. Mildred is vexed with us for permitting all this banging, and we have put the box away carefully in the attic. It is too early to judge results, but the outlook is hopeful. One of our colleagues has just rung Anatomy and obtained the Post-mortem room, which is at least a near miss, and the epidiascope, after sulking for three weeks, is now working feverishly, and has set fire to a picture of Percivall Pott.

Professorial Chair

SINCE the man from the Ministry fell through the seat of our Senior Lecturer's chair some time ago the University has been turning over in its mind the desirability of allowing us to purchase some new chairs. The green light came last month, and we have all been breathlessly awaiting the arrival of our new Professorial Chair. Our Professor is not a man to throw away an opportunity of getting a decent seat for the first time in his medical career, and he has been happily studying the form in several highly coloured catalogues. On sordid financial grounds he was regretfully forced to leave out of consideration the 'Floating-Eez' (at the touch of a button instantly assumes any angle desired; the business man's dream; guaranteed for a lifetime), and the Executive's Chair (padded arm-rests and stout swivel mechanism; a solid job) seemed lacking in dignity. The Director's Chair (with foam-rubber seat and adjustable back; in blue, red, or green) was rather better, but our efficient administrator, who rules us in aesthetic matters, maintained that in her opinion the rest of the furnishings were not suited to admixture with primary colours. There was accordingly little choice in the matter, and our accommodating Professor was driven to turn his mind to those chairs which were obtainable in pastel shades.

Fortunately the Chairman's Chair (with foam-rubber seat, stout swivel mechanism, *and* patent adjustable tilting mechanism) came in grey or black, and this morning a grey one arrived in the hall, swathed in paper padding and secured at all points with string. We tiptoed cautiously round it, exploring the foam rubber, and examining the tilting mechanism; rather enviously we watched it borne away into the professorial sanctum. But mark the sequel.

It appears that our Professor was hospitably entertaining the Vice-Chancellor at morning tea when he conceived the injudicious notion of putting the Chairman's Chair through its paces for the benefit of his guest. The first tentative circuit of the stout swivel caused him to crack his patella viciously on a totally unexpected corner of his desk, and while expressing himself with some force on this occurrence he unwisely leant backwards, thereby bringing into play the patent adjustable tilting mechanism to such effect that the whole chair, complete with Professor, overbalanced backwards, causing him to strike his head a savage blow on the corner of the bookcase. The Vice-Chancellor's tea spilled all over the desk and overflowed on to his trousers, and our gallant administrator, roused by the clatter, tripped over the mat on the way to the rescue and joined the chaos on the floor.

The Chairman's Chair is now in the possession of our stolid Senior Lecturer, and our Professor has taken over a wooden affair which used to stand in the room where the cleaners make their tea.

Noise Pollution

AN atypical surgical friend of ours is by nature a placid, easy-going type, addicted to peace and quiet—we have sometimes wondered if his thyroid might be mildly inadequate. Not for him the red mist in front of the eyes, the broken golfclub, the bitten carpet. All the time we have known him he has never thrown a scalpel at the theatre sister except under extreme provocation. Our friend has recently relinquished clinical life in favour of the sequestered calm of the University, and when we met him the other day we expected to find him more than usually urbane. But not so; his eyes were shifty and his fingers twitched.

It appears that one day last week a chap arrived with a pneumatic drill to tear up some concrete flooring next door to our friend's lab. No-one had thought to warn him of the impending cataclysm, and the initial burst of the drill caused him to rise three feet in the air, completely severing the terminal portion of his tongue. By the time he grounded again, some distance from take-off, the entire lab. was vibrating, and for the rest of the morning important telephone messages were blasted out of existence, consecutive thought was rendered impossible, and our friend was thrown about in his chair like a pea in a bottle. At 2.10 p.m. the man went home, and our friend's eardrums twanged in heartfelt relief.

At 2.15 p.m. precisely a gigantic sanding machine began to operate in the passage outside. Our friend tells us that the vibration dislodged two fillings in his teeth and sent several thermostats demented. In vain did he attempt to reason with the operator, who had his orders and insisted on carrying them out. However, after two hours the epicentre gradually receded into the distance; our friend took a refreshing draught of amylobarbitone and settled down to work.

Seven and a quarter minutes later a brightly coloured truck dashed round the corner and came to rest under the window. Two large men leaped out and began to fiddle with a complex engine mounted on the back; immediately a thunderous rubbing noise burst forth from the bowels of the machine. Our friend's room began to move to and fro; reprints fell like ticker-tape from the shelves, pictures swayed and rattled, and the desk edged itself across the floor towards the window. Our friend staggered out to enquire from the Secretary what was going on. 'It *is* a nasty noise, isn't it?' screamed the Secretary brightly, in a wild British understatement; 'I do wish the Botany department would sterilise their flowerpots somewhere else!'

Every man has his breaking-point. Our friend reached for the telephone with a trembling hand and dialled the Professor of Botany. After a brief sketch of his views on the history and technique of flowerpot sterilisation he adumbrated his opinion of the character, morals, and antecedents of the operators and of the motives which prompted them to undertake flowerpot sterilisation outside his window rather than outside the Botany department.

The next day all was peace, but in the heat of his one great moment he omitted to remember that the Professor of Botany is also the acting Vice-Chancellor. Our friend is now waiting, an apprehensive and broken man, to be stripped of his academic buttons.

Active Learning

OUR lecture room exemplifies the British ideal of the maximum of inaudibility with the minimum of ventilation. The seating is carefully designed so that the knees of the student become painfully and inextricably wedged against the sharp edge of the bench in front, while the spines of his scapulae are assailed by the sharp edge of the bench behind. The occupants of the back benches, out of earshot and almost out of sight of authority, spend their time happily playing pontoon. In contrast, the seekers after truth in the first two rows either gaze soulfully at the lecturer's face, their lips moving silently to the rhythm of his discourse, or feverishly attempt to record in their notebooks every word and every significant cough or pause in the hope that it will come up in the exam.

In the middle rows between these two extremes is the great student body, vast, inchoate, and drowsy. When one of its legs goes to sleep it painfully shifts round on to the other, and when darkness falls it gratefully closes its eyes to the slides and scratches its itchy places. It is not learning, it is not even listening, it is merely indulging the herd instinct and a sense of cosy companionship in the dark. It is this middle section we have long desired to reach. We are paid to communicate our experience to these young minds, to lay our burden of knowledge at their feet, to pass on the torch. Till now our oratory, our sarcasm, our highly polished witticisms, and our depth of erudition have alike failed to project our personality beyond the front row. At last, however, we have found the answer.

In a recent number of *Family Doctor* some exhilarating experiments are reported in which university students were given words to memorise. Without warning the light went out, the backs of their chairs fell off and the arms became electrified. In addition a revolver was fired and a sheet of iron fell to the floor. This is the technique for us. 'Mark my words!', we shall roar. 'You sir, at the end of the fourteenth row, what have I just been saying?' And as we press the appropriate button the floor of his seat will give way, a bucket of water will fall on his head, and he will automatically be precipitated down the gangway to our feet. 'Let this be a lesson to you, sir' we shall say sternly, as we speed him back to his place with a well-aimed revolver bullet. It beats us why we didn't think of it before.

Teaching by Taste

NOW that we are reconsidering the details of our medical course we feel that we should take every opportunity of giving our students a wide knowledge of the inter-relationships of medicine and modern society. A conducted tour of the local brewery is an accepted feature of the class in microbiology in many medical schools, but here we can go one better, for we are on excellent terms, not only with the local brewery, but also with one of the local vignerons, and our enthusiastic microbiologist has already inserted tours of both establishments into the syllabus. On each the exposition is followed by a judicious sampling of the products in rooms thoughtfully provided for the purpose. Only by field-work of this kind, it is felt, will the students acquire a proper respect for the name of Pasteur and an understanding of the basic importance of microbiology. Not only this, but our socially conscious Professor of Medicine considers it vital that the students should gain some insight into the problems of alcoholism, and feels that this might best be provided by a second visit to the vineyards—a visit on which the conversation would take a very different turn, though the final sampling procedure would be almost identical.

Now the surgeons, in their bluff way, would like to take their tutorial classes along for a historical chat on the use of wine as a surgical antiseptic, and even our pathologist thinks he would find it convenient to expound upon cirrhosis surrounded by a supply of the causative agent. In such an atmosphere we have been forced to meditate on the possibility of making use of these unrivalled facilities for the benefit of preclinical students. It has been urged, for example, that our lectures on the mechanisms of swallowing might be supplemented by practical work in the field, or that a class on reaction-times could be profitably arranged. We ourselves see no need to advance such specious arguments, for we well remember an educational experience we had some years ago, when the medical society of which we were then a member invited a director of a wine firm to guide us through a small selection of his wares.

The wines were ranged in line on a white-covered table, with reinforcements underneath. The society gazed solemnly through the glasses at the guttering candles provided, it inhaled the aroma up the backs of its noses, and for the first three bottles or thereabouts it spat out the mouthfuls into a bucket in professional style. But when it came to one it liked, the discipline broke down, and by the time it reached the sixth or seventh bottle it was drinking heartily. Afterwards we were surprised to find that our ranking of the first four was identical with that of the society's impresario, though our vocabulary was not in his class. For example, what we had said about the Châteauneuf-du-Pape 1947 was 'alpha minus; taste good, colour good, smell good'. What we should have said was 'A noticeable burnt, roasted flavour; a very good glass of wine'. Of the winner, a

Corton 1928, our notes read: 'alpha; very pleasant'. This, we found, was 'A beautiful glass of wine, lacking the astringent pull of young wine. Lovely smooth soft drinking, with a wonderful breeding and bouquet. The finest drink on the slab'. Of the Fleurie 1950, which was last in order of sampling, we had written, in handwriting by this time grown rather large and expansive: 'Undistinguished'. Clearly we had begun to find our form, but what we had really meant was: 'A hard, unyielding, unforthcoming wine, a little harsh on the nose'.

It seems obvious to us that an organised wine-tasting is in itself an excellent educative procedure to include in the pre-clinical curriculum. It would develop all those qualities which the clinicians find deficient in our students – their command of language, their powers of observation and description, and their capacity to synthesise information and come to a decision. We are bringing the matter to the notice of the Faculty tomorrow.

The Great Escape

WE heard an alarming tale the other day from a friend of ours whose duty and pleasure it is to remove one of the more inaccessible supernumerary organs with which the human body is so temptingly equipped. It seems that he had thought of a new approach to his accustomed prize, and so it came about that he found himself one afternoon alone in the dissecting-room with an assortment of anatomical bits and pieces on which to map his course. After a time the dictates of Nature interrupted his engrossing task and caused our friend to retire to the lavatory at the far end of the room; unfortunately his withdrawal coincided with the arrival of the dissecting-room attendant to lock up. Seeing nobody inside, the attendant concluded that our friend had gone home, whereupon he locked the doors and repaired to his tea.

Like most surgeons, our friend is a quick thinker, and when he discovered his situation it was at once clear to him that he must get out. He banged and shouted for some time without result; anatomists find the study of anatomy no longer tolerable at a fairly early hour, and the building appeared to be deserted. Suppressing the surgical language which rose to his lips, our friend made the circuit of his prison. Except for a large cupboard in one corner, the walls were smooth and unbroken; the room was lit from the roof. It occurred to him that he might pile one table on another and so reach freedom, but the tables were bolted to the floor. It was about this time that he first observed a narrow metal rod actuating a roof-ventilator, but he rejected the idea with a shudder. However, after the passage of a further half-hour, during which our friend banged intermittently, he conceived an unreasoning distaste for the illustrations with which the room was illiberally furnished, and so forced himself to consider the ventilator seriously. The climb was one of some fifteen feet, and our friend has left behind the carefree rapture of his student days in the gym. However, after a nightmare journey during which his pinstriped trousers were irretrievably ruined and his intervertebral discs maimed for life, he clambered precariously through the ventilator on to a dangerous ledge, to the great astonishment of the Secretary to the department of Anthropology, who courteously assisted him to climb in through her window and rejoin the rest of humanity by means of her staircase.

Our friend made something of the story at dinner that night, touching lightly on the well-known psychogenic effects of a night spent in a dissecting-room, dwelling momentarily on the dangers of his escape, and including an entirely ethical disclaimer of any special skill or ability. It was not until the next day that he discovered that what he had taken for a cupboard was the automatic elevator used for the bodies, which would have taken him straight down to the basement, a telephone and freedom.

Simultaneous Translation

IT is a cross which I am becoming accustomed to bear that after all these years of public speaking I am still not a Public Speaker. Not for me the polished orotundities, the yeasty metaphor, the effortless scintillation. My slightest public utterances are preceded by days of malaise in which my sluggish wits mumble together, and the oratorical pearls of preceding speakers pass unheeded through my thudding eardrums. As the fatal moment arrives when the chairman calls upon Doctor, ah, Doctor, um . . . to deliver his paper on (here he peers closely at the agenda) . . . to deliver his paper—the witches broth produced by my tormented adrenals deprives all but my hypothalamus of its function.

All this is a legitimate occupational hazard; one cannot make a congress without breaking a few addled eggs. I am used to it all now: the commiserating glance of my neighbour as I return to my seat, the convulsive clapping of those awakened by the commotion, and the ghastly silence when the chairman calls for a discussion of the most valuable and interesting paper to which we have just had the pleasure of listening. But at the World Conference last week I plumbed a further depth of degradation; I was Simultaneously Translated.

To a man who is virtually a pithed preparation when he stands up to speak, there is something curiously unnerving in knowing that when he mutters a dehydrated 'Mr. Chairman, Ladies and Gentlemen' into a microphone—enough in itself to appal the stoutest heart—what reaches his audience may well be '¡Señor Presidente, Señoras y Señores!' impeccably enunciated in a clear high feminine voice. Nor does the certainty that three-quarters of the audience have switched over to the French version to improve their accent and that the remainder are fiddling with the apparatus in the hope of getting Radio 1, steady his mind for the peroration. His Little Jokes congeal on his tongue as he realises they are untranslatable, and in the ensuing confusion colloquialisms and slang rise tumbling to his lips till the red light mercifully cuts them off. Meanwhile the tape recorders grind majestically on, enshrining his part in the proceedings for his children's children.

Perhaps it is all to the good. At least I know what a United Nation feels like.

Urogenic Index

SOME years ago we attended a World Conference on Medical Education, and since then we have taken our teaching very seriously indeed. In the bosom of our family we are constantly accused of speaking through our teeth or mumbling into the paper, so that the crystal clarity of our thought processes often fails to communicate itself to the assembled company. It occurred to us that our students might labour under the same handicap, and that our aphorisms, which echo so pleasantly in our accessory sinuses, might perhaps become somewhat dulled or blunted in their passage through our dentures to the atmosphere of the lecture room. It being impossible to obtain any direct information on this point (through long practice our students wear exactly the same expressions whether they are awake or asleep), we have cast about for some objective way of assessing the audience reaction to our lectures, so that we might compare their effect with the reactions produced by our colleagues. We are always too flustered to make an accurate count of those who have to be nudged back to consciousness when we stop, and a preliminary trial convinced us that neither the number of coughs nor the number of coins dropped on the floor during our discourse was a suitable index. In the circumstances we have finally settled on an indirect technique.

In New York, the reaction to a television programme used sometimes to be measured by the flow of water discharged into the sewers of the city at its conclusion, the figure obtained being known as the 'teleflush rating' of the programme. We have no flowmeter adaptable for this purpose, but are confident that a tape recorder installed in conjunction with a suitable amplifier in relation to the main outlet pipe of the department would afford substantially the same information. By dividing the duration of the recorded disturbance by the number of students attending the lecture we should be able to arrive at a figure representing student opinion with some accuracy. We propose that this figure be known as the urogenic index, and at the next World Conference we shall publish our preliminary results.

The Prodigal Son

ABOUT this time of the year we begin to have trouble with our exchange scholars and travel grantees who have just got back from the States. We do not refer, of course, to those simple souls who come back with a 3D sweater girl bulging at the lower end of their ties ('Strictly for Laughs'), or with a pair of luminous socks ('They Shine in the Dark; One Red, One Blue'). Nor do we mean the more complex personalities who offer us cigarettes ('King-size this side, Regular the other'), or start convulsively and say 'You're welcome' at inappropriate moments. Our friends are cast in a more subtle mould; the trouble goes deeper than this. In the restaurant they embarrass us by asking for the Sea Food Menu and declining coffee with a delicate shudder. They spend fruitless moments looking for Channel 7 on our television set, they ask for donuts with a slight emphasis on the elided letters, and they even use coat-hangers in their cars.

This sort of thing reached its height in one of our own department's returnees, a hitherto rather colourless scientific type, who was discovered the other day absently wandering round the basement looking for the 'Coca-Cola' machine. It was after we had found him staring at a pound-note in a puzzled way and complaining that it wouldn't go into his bill-fold that we gave up trying to take no notice. 'Tell us,' we begged, 'tell us about America.' The resulting session has left us in an apprehensive state, and we have placed ourselves in quarantine as a precaution. When our friend thanked us for our attention we replied, to our horror, 'You bet', and since then symptoms are developing rapidly. Only this morning we had an impulse to put up a notice saying 'Think' over our bench.

Humane Anatomist

AN acquaintance of ours, a hard-bitten irascible anatomist who is reputed to eat ignorant first-year students for breakfast, recently had occasion to change his newsagent. When the bill came it was addressed to him at the department of Humane Anatomy. Since this tribute he has not been the same man. Our spies report that yesterday when someone was not attending in the osteology class he threw a humerus at the offender, though the femur was ready to his hand, and this morning he let a student through his viva on the infratemporal fossa first shot.

Furniture Removing

A scientific friend of ours had occasion recently to attend a meeting in one of the brisk industrial cities of the North, and was offered accommodation in a women's hostel. Ever anxious to see how the other half lives, our friend accepted; and it is a tribute to his scientific spirit that he persevered even on finding that the female denizens were still in residence.

He was a trifle mystified to find in his room a notice saying 'No furniture is to be removed from this room without permission of the warden', but it came to him that the midnight-feast tradition of his own schooldays might be represented among the female sex by midnight furniture-removing parties. The hormones, you know. He was, however, fascinated to find similar notices on the top of the bookcase and on the back of the wardrobe. The room was dark and damp, and surrounded on all sides by a stand of sturdy rhubarb. However, the high holiday spirits common to all whose expenses have been paid carried him through until bedtime, when he first took adequate stock of the sleeping apparatus provided.

Our friend is a large man, and like so many large men nowadays (and for that matter small women too) he suffers from a Disc. The bed had been designed for an achondroplasic some four feet in length, and a large iron bar had been placed at either end to prevent the achondroplasic from pushing her feet or her head beyond the allotted span. It was now too late to make representations, and there was nothing for it but to sleep on the floor. The bedding came off reluctantly, exposing a by now familiar notice on the bedstead.

Our friend spent an uneasy night. The stairs re-echoed to the sound of girlish laughter until after midnight, and in a room across the rhubarb a furniture-removing party was in progress. He was able to stem the torrents of light and sound flowing through the fanlight with a blanket, and, flushed with success, attempted a similar operation on the window, a pane of which promptly fell out with a thunderous crash into the rhubarb. Our friend waited timorously for the Head Girl, but no-one took any notice; clearly windows did not come under the furniture-removing ban.

At two the owls took over, rooting mournfully about in the rhubarb outside the space where the window had been. Our friend is something of an ornithologist, and recognised every known British species as well as a number of South American families. The floor was hard, and so were the osteophytes in his lumbar spine. Moreover, there were several pieces of scrap metal in his pillow, and at half past four he gave it up and concentrated on his Simenon.

There were no mirrors in the bathroom—so much for feminine vanity—and our friend shaved guiltily by his reflection in the door-knob, not daring to remove the mirror from his room without first approaching the warden. After breakfast he left as hurriedly as possible, having first signed himself in on the visitors' book as a male guest of the Head Girl on the previous evening and carefully omitted to sign himself out again.

Dust

A statistical colleague of ours—a fastidious man—recently complained about the dust which persistently collected in his room. By a series of experiments involving the analysis of variance and the closing of different windows and doors he had been able to exclude both the corridor and the road outside as possible sources. His room was regularly cleaned, and he had had it hermetically sealed, but still the dust advanced, grey, cosmic, menacing. He wished, he said, he had some means of determining the nature of the deposit; it might, he hinted, be extraplanetary in origin, or due to the activities of a mathematically inclined poltergeist.

An appeal of this nature could not be ignored, and within ten minutes a battery of microscopes had been set up, and the mantles of Sherlock Holmes and Dr. Thorndyke had descended upon us. With watch glasses and camel-hair brushes we crawled under the tables, labelling each specimen carefully with the precise source and date. With glad cries we attracted each other's attention: 'Quick, Watson, the Coley's fluid!' 'What do you make of this rotifer, Jarvis?' 'Undoubtedly the hair of a camel, my dear Watson.' 'Extraordinary, my dear Holmes!' 'But very elementary.'

We investigated the turn-ups of our colleague's trousers and the contents of the breast-pocket of his lab-coat; we spent a happy hour devising miniature dust-extractors. The bubble burst when tea arrived and we leant back exhausted, our gaze seeking inspiration in the ceiling. Even as we watched, a crack appeared and a little trickle of extraplanetary dust floated down to settle on our colleague's microcomputer.

Swell Gals

RUMMAGING in my superannuated files the other day I found the suggested texts which Western Union used to put out in the 1950s for the benefit of busy executives or inarticulate teenagers who had neither the time nor the ability to think up a message of their own when confronted with a special occasion. All the sender had to do was to tick the message which appealed to him and Western Union, after its palm had been crossed with silver, did the rest. Next to the rubrics for Mother's Day (sample: 'To Mother a thousand kisses. Hope that not a single one misses') was the sheet for Secretaries Day, a festival which has never gained a great deal of ground on this side of the Atlantic. Perhaps I have been remiss in not wording my secretaries up with: 'On Secretaries Day and every day, you're tops with us in every way. Best of everything to a swell gal.'

On the other hand, perhaps not. Not all my geese have been swans, and one who regularly reported sick when any departmental crisis was at hand deserved no fulsome commendation. Nor did another whose spelling centre had been selectively obliterated by an otherwise silent cerebral catastrophe. Even the swans (of which there were several) presented some difficulties. One of them had been secretary to a British Cabinet Minister before casting in her lot with me, and to address her in this way would have smacked of lèse majesté. And my last secretary was graded as an administrative assistant; I feel that to substitute Administrative Assistant's Day in the messages provided would adversely affect their metre. But none of this diminishes my sincere regard for the difficult job they all did, and now that I am my own secretary I am happy to pay them a belated tribute.

Fashion Class

Most anatomists eke out a meagre livelihood by distilling the essence of their subject to improbable groups of people, and in common with many of my fellows I teach anatomy to art students. For some time the class and I have felt that all was not well. Now at last I have put my finger on the reason—this purely representational stuff is getting us nowhere. Next year I am to start a course in Commercial Anatomy for Fashion Illustrators, thus at one stroke raising myself above the ruck into the realms of a possible distinction award and offering to my class the chance of eventually earning a living.

The course will concentrate on fundamentals: we shall start with the Evidences of Structural Adaptation to Haute Couture. Under this heading we shall deal with the Atretic Waist, the Pinhole Nostril, the Double-jointed Digit, and the High Centre of Gravity. We shall pass to the Relationships Between Bodily Proportions and Artistic Media. In this section comes the discussion on the correlation of relative head length with the glossiness of the paper expressed in reflectivity units, and the account of the Expanding or Telescopic Thigh, with notes on the peak values of thigh length obtained in half-tone blocks advertising nylons. There will be a lecture on o.s. illustrating, with a word on the Bosom, and some remarks on the Undistributed Middle. The course will end with a discussion on Commercial Postural Equilibrium, with a subsection dealing with the use of the Shooting Stick.

Entries are already being received: *make sure of your booking NOW.*

Ancient Mariner

There is something about retiring from an academic post which tends to release a flood of garrulity. One of my colleagues, who recently became an emeritus, retains a room in his department for research purposes, and now joins his erstwhile staff for morning coffee and afternoon tea. Such is the flow of reminiscence and anecdote at these sessions that the work of the department has begun to suffer. As a result a roster has had to be instituted whereby every day one staff member is deputed to act as audience while the others escape to their various duties. The listener on duty is charged to be adequately receptive, swearing the while in faith 'twas strange, 'twas passing strange, 'twas pitiful, 'twas wondrous pitiful.

A different emeritus prowls the corridors of the hospital and, like the Ancient Mariner, stoppeth one of three in order to discourse on the days when the hospital (and indeed the world) was young. It is occasionally possible to accelerate and pass him at speed, waving a greeting expressive of an extremely urgent mission. However, this rarely succeeds, and the safer procedure is to port or starboard the helm up the nearest side corridor. This often makes landfall for the navigator in unfamiliar territory, such as Podiatry or the Appliances Store, where he may be at something of a loss to account for his visit.

Such phenomena may be the aftermath of lives spent in listening to the histories of patients; for too many years words have been pent up without a suitable outlet. My own retirement life style provides no captive audience, and I am reduced to talking either to my dog or to myself. For the most part I do not find this distressing, for I have always been highly introverted, but I sometimes feel that my experiences deserve to reach a wider and more appreciative public. Perhaps I might hire the village hall and get some of them off my chest.

Serendipity

THE media constantly seek to persuade us that the best scientific discoveries are those which result from fortunate accidents. Archimedes and his bath, Galvani and his frogs' legs, Roentgen and his photographic plate, Fleming and his contaminated cultures—all these remind them of Walpole's tale of the three princes of Serendip, who were 'always making discoveries, by accident and sagacity, of things they were not in quest of'.

But what the media do not stress is the unfortunate position of those scientists who have not had an appropriate accident. Like me, for instance. For many years now I have been awaiting a felicitous mishap, but still it does not come. I do not seem to be adequately accident-prone, and such accidents as I do have are never of the right kind. When one of my rats is found dead, it is never of a virus disease unknown to microbiology, but only because it struck up an argument with a rat bigger than itself. If the power supply fails in the middle of one of my experiments, it does not reveal activity in a new system of nerve fibres; it simply delivers 240 volts through my finger and thumb when it comes on again. If the tissue I am investigating is put into the wrong solution by mistake I do not discover a new approach to superconductivity, I simply get a squashy mess. In short, I have little in common as regards accidents with the princes of Serendip.

Nor can I compete with their sagacity. Pasteur is reputed to have said (no doubt in French), 'Fortune favours the prepared mind', and I am obliged to confess that my mind is no longer so well prepared as it once was. Nowadays it lies down comfortably when not whipped into action, and cannot be relied on to hunt on its own. If I go to bed with a problem on my mind I do not wake up with the solution; I wake up with a sore head. Unlike many fortunate beings, I cannot concentrate on one thing while doing another. When I paint the trellis my mind is fully occupied with painting the trellis, and is unable to reach out to encompass the solution of scientific, or indeed domestic, difficulties. Perhaps I am not really a scientist at all. Such a man deserves no accident, no serendipity. Yet I still hope.

Medical Catering

AN academic friend of ours recently took up an appointment in postgraduate education in a new and shiny hospital. The educational part of his job presented no problems, but nothing had prepared him for his catering responsibilities. Like so many institutions, shiny or otherwise, the hospital was in the grip of a ferocious economy drive, and the administration demanded a precise forecast of the quantity and quality of the food to be made available at every form of postgraduate education, from small working lunches to enormous showpieces involving overseas visitors. Ordering too much led to painful interviews with the catering officer, who was sneakily prone to refer the matter to the bluff and outspoken accountant; ordering too little led to painful interviews with latecomers (usually bluff and outspoken surgeons) who had arrived to find nothing more than a few tattered scraps of lettuce and some fragments of cheese.

But after a few months our friend began to get the hang of it, and felt confident enough to specify exotic provender on special occasions. Perhaps inevitably, this led to disaster when, on an invitation to an important evening reception for a visiting professor, he omitted to mention that food would be featured, so that the majority of the audience arrived having already eaten.

Our friend found himself at 11 p.m. in charge of some 3 kg of devilled prawns, several large platters of chicken Vichy and beef and mushroom stew, unheard of quantities of stuffed eggs and sandwiches, and some bowls of fruit salad. He could find no one anxious to collaborate in a free midnight feast, so he stowed most of the detritus into the administration refrigerator, intending to dispose of it early next morning among his friends in the secretariat. In this he was unfortunately frustrated by the even earlier arrival of the accountant, who had explored the refrigerator for milk to take with his coffee.

The resulting painful interview was a masterpiece of its kind, and our friend now sticks to fish and chips or sandwiches for evening functions, no matter how fashionable the current visitor may be.

Evolution of Examiners

A colleague of ours whose whim it is to act as external examiner recently took part in some rather sordid anatomy vivas. Outside the door of the fatal room, in the corridor where his victims congregated, were several illustrations and a family tree designed to stimulate an interest in the ancestry and zoological relationships of Man. Having completed their savage work, he and his co-examiner emerged blinking to find something faintly unfamiliar about the outside world. Closer investigation revealed an addition to the family tree made by sticking adhesive paper to the glass. There, on one of the main trunks, between Eoanthropus and Australopithecus, was a new branch bearing the single word *Examiners*.

Advice to Examinees

FOR a generation now I have been consulted by students anxious to know how best to plan the defeat of the examiners at the end of the year. I have never known what general advice to give them, for in my ignorance I believed that every man is an individual, and must adopt individual methods in order to succeed. But a friend of mine who is taking a degree in education has provided me with the solution which was solemnly laid down for him by his mentors: 'Organise your knowledge at the recall level.' I have been telling this slogan to all my students this year, with the offer of a small prize to anybody who can tell me what the advice means, and a further prize to those who can tell me how to follow it.

Halcyon Weeks

FOR me, this is the best time of the year—the halcyon weeks just before the exams, when the students start to bend at the hips as I pass them in the corridors. Naturally, this has nothing to do with the fact that I am the internal examiner; it just happens that about this time of the term their innate good manners come to the surface. For the rest of the year these are fairly well submerged, and there is a regrettable tendency to elbow Sir aside at the local cinema, if he is constituting an obstruction on the way to the ice-cream, or to pay his witticisms less than their due meed of attention. But for this fortnight nothing is too good for me; my jokes are all excellent, my arrival hushes all comment. If I drop something in the tutorial class, at least three people collide with each other in their efforts to help me to regain possession of my property. It is all most soothing.

After the exams, of course, the trouble starts—the letters from Mum and Dad, the interviews, the post-mortems, the medical certificates, the tales of horrifying mischance, the fatherly advice, the promises of reform, the choice of alternative careers. But by then I have had my fortnight, and fate cannot touch me.

College of Medical Examiners

EXTERNAL examiners are often cynical men, who affect to be able to mark a candidate accurately from the first paragraph of his paper or from an inspection of his finger-nails. It is, however, clearly desirable that they should be versed in the theory and practice of examining in order that they may present a façade of judicious impartiality towards the candidate. The College of Medical Examiners and its affiliated body, the Chartered Society of Licensed Invigilators, have been founded to standardise the accomplishments of examiners in this respect. At present the college offers two diplomas: the membership enables its possessor to examine for the various qualifying degrees and diplomas, while the fellowship is necessary for examiners aspiring to higher things. It is intended shortly to institute a third diploma, that of tropical examining (D.T.E.), but the syllabus for this diploma has not yet been fully approved by the court.

The diploma of fellow is granted only for outstanding contributions to the science of examining, such as the raising of the failure-rate in the Conjoint to 80%, or the introduction of pin-striped trousers and a stand-up collar to a Biochemistry viva.

The syllabus for the membership includes the theory of ambiguous questions, the elucidation of hieroglyphic writings and the Rorschach interpretation of ink blots, the effects of adrenaline on the speech centre, the use and abuse of sarcasm, and the care and retention of the mark sheet. Candidates are also required to undergo a practical and viva voce examination at which their reactions to bad spelling, dirty collars and unshaven faces will be assessed. The following is a specimen paper:

COLLEGE OF MEDICAL EXAMINERS

PRIMARY EXAMINATION FOR THE DIPLOMA OF MEMBERSHIP

Human Anatomy

Time allowed: 3 hours. Not more than *six* questions to be attempted.

1. A candidate appears for his viva voce examination wearing spats. Outline the steps you would take to deal with the situation, giving your reasons.
2. Identify (*a*) the seraphic vein; (*b*) the abducter tubercal; (*c*) the vegetable pole; (*d*) the accessory do; (*e*) the anteroposterior surface of the ileum; (*f*) the uterine ossicles.
3. Enumerate the methods used to give the impression of immense knowledge frustrated by writer's cramp, other than the basic 'Sorry, no time.'
4. Illustrate the following situations by clearly labelled diagrams:

   (*a*) 'The bursar lying between the two joints is often fenestrated.'
   (*b*) 'The kidney excretes the surplice.'

5. Write a short essay on the ball-point pen.
6. What did the candidate have in mind when he wrote the following:

   (*a*) 'a capsular joint with an articulating capsule in the joint cavity.'
   (*b*) 'these bones are concerned with maintaining body stature.'
   (*c*) 'the uterus turns inside out and there you are.'

Deceitful Examiners

DURING my working life I never gave advice unless I was asked for it, but now I have retired I have begun to reconsider this attitude. As you grow older, your illusions are progressively stripped away, but some are backed by stronger adhesive than others, and the most tenacious of all is the illusion that you have some advice worth passing on. (The penultimate one to fall off is, of course, the illusion that somebody may actually *take* this advice.)

I have therefore been casting around for a maxim which might reverberate throughout posterity. Many others are already current, such as those put about by Perelman: 'Never play cards with a man called Doc; never eat at a place called Mom's; never sleep with anyone whose troubles are greater than your own'.

In academic medicine the most useful one is: 'Never run after a bus, a woman, or a new educational theory; there will be another one along in a moment'. I should like to add another maxim to operate in this particular field.

One of the most formative experiences of my life occurred at the age of six, when a teacher asked us how we breathed during the day. One of my colleagues ventured the opinion that we breathed through our noses. 'Excellent', she said, 'and now, how do we breathe during the night?' Clearly something different was demanded, and I bravely said that we breathed through our mouths. (I was fairly sure of this, for such was my own adenoidal practice). To my consternation the answer was no, we breathed at night exactly as we breathed during the day. I was appalled. That this woman, who had seemed entirely trustworthy, should double-cross me in this fashion was intolerable, and I burst smartly into tears. But I received an indelible lesson, and from that moment on I suspected that every examination question I was asked might have been designed to mislead innocent examinees.

In the 82 examinations inflicted on me during my medical education I bore this principle successfully in mind, but when I became an examiner myself I tried to ensure that every question I asked was honestly phrased and devoid of traps.

Nowadays, when I look through the dodgy 'true or false' questions which determine the course of medical careers, it sometimes seems to me that honesty is dead, and the advice I should like to bequeath to humanity is simply this: 'Never trust an examiner'.

Alternative Careers

AS examiners grow senile and contemplative they tend to meditate on the fate of their examinees. What happens to all these characters who think that megakaryocytes form the white matter of the cerebral hemispheres, or that the decidua basalis is part of the sensory system of the tongue? The other night we wished we had an adequate follow-up service, so that we could write a statistical paper on it, with five-year survival rates and incomprehensible little tables scattered throughout the text. We remembered one chap who was for a time wont to fence with us across the examiners' table, and ultimately became private secretary to a maharajah, and another who joined the Foreign Legion. Another is happily printing Christmas cards, and one of our earliest victims is designing computers. It seems to us that too little attention is paid to this kind of thing, and that as a profession we ought to investigate the careers for which failure in our examinations particularly suits a man.

At this point our speculations were cut short by a knock on our door and the entry of an old friend – a veteran of several gallant skirmishes with anatomy and physiology, and a victim of the wholly unreasonable demands of pathology. We asked him what he was doing now, and he told us he was driving a soft drinks lorry through the North of England. 'As a matter of fact', he said, 'I've got the old bus outside.' We peeped through the curtains, and there, sure enough, was a gigantic lorry. 'Seven thousand bottles', said our friend proudly, and we had to believe him.

Tea Club

OUR tea club is an old and respected institution. The tea is manufactured from two vast kettles in a picturesque array of teapots in the subterranean cavern in the basement, and is distributed by safe hand on trays to the parched occupants of the periphery of the building. It is our experience, however, that the safer the hand the slower the feet, and by the time the third storey is reached not a few of the original calories have escaped into the circumambient atmosphere. Further, during the vicissitudes of the journey the destination of the cups, originally crystal clear, becomes sullied with uncertainty, so that the member at the end of the round never knows whether he is to receive a cup bearing the inscription 'Lab. 5', 'Cleaners', or, more simply, 'Peggy.' The other day we were interested to find ourselves drinking out of a cup with the stark label 'Rat linseed'.

In 1939 the iron hand of war reached down into our basement and dealt the tea club a blow from which it has never fully recovered. Even now the sugar gives out towards the middle of the third week of the ration period, and those of us who are accustomed to protect our livers from the effects of tannic-acid absorption by the judicious ingestion of sucrose spend an unhappy few days. Our genial and courteous Animal Man is occasionally in a position to alleviate our distress by impounding—without their knowledge or permission—some of the monkeys' sugar. During the Black Days he frequently brings in a lump with the comforting assurance: 'It's all right, sir, they'll never miss it.'

In the circumstances, however, it is not surprising that there should be mutterings among those who are not placed so fortunately adjacent to the animal house, and a splinter group has actually been formed to drink illicit coffee. They post lookouts in the corridors, and their source of carbohydrate is a jealously guarded secret, but it is suspected that much is due to their foresight in co-opting a visiting American. Once a week we have a departmental tea-party, at which both the orthodox and the seceders partake of cake; and our conscientious accountant has worked out the fraction of the tea-club subscription which non-members have to pay to qualify for two slices. Even so, unscrupulous dissenters have been observed lingering behind after the party is over to pick up a few crumbs which they have not paid for. Feeling runs high, especially as it is has recently been found necessary to raise the subscription, and it is felt that a stand should be taken on the matter. Since the recent cold spell, however, we have lost our confidence that a stand would be successful, for there are indications of disunity in the highest places. Twice in one week our President-Secretary-Treasurer has been discovered guiltily drinking 'Bovril.'

Ernie's Winter

IN our department we don't worry about calendars or solstices or any new-fangled nonsense like that: our winter begins when Ernie says it does. Ernie is the chap who works the furnace, and the only man who understands our complicated heating system. If we are in early enough on the great day we are privileged to hear a tone-poem in sound. A vast roaring noise begins somewhere in the basement and gradually builds up into a high-pitched scream as it sweeps its way through the lower reaches of the building. By the time it has reached the lab below our eyrie the pipes around our wall have started to shake with excitement, and the scream gives way to a series of titanic hammer-blows which lift our typewriter off its perch and send our reprints flying. Eventually the tumult quietens to a steady ticking noise, and when we stretch our legs under our bench we find that the radiator is red hot. Winter has come.

This time, however, winter did not come so smoothly as usual. The hammer-blows stopped on the second storey, and our radiator remained obstinately cold. We felt it necessary to inform Ernie of the hitch in his plans, and he honoured us with a personal visit. The consultation left us a trifle uneasy. It appeared that there was cement in one of the valves controlling our radiator, and it was a miracle that we had not blown up long ago. Ernie retired to the basement to shut off winter while the affected valve was dealt with, and when he came back we got under the bench with him to inspect the outrage. It was then that we noticed another valve on the pipe, hidden in an inaccessible corner, and asked Ernie what it was for. 'Oh,' said Ernie carelessly, 'that's a by-pass for Biochemistry; you're first on the circuit here, and if that's shut they get no heating.'

This dangerous information has been in our possession for some time now, and our baser impulses are simmering. We have a spanner from the workshop in our drawer, and only yesterday the Professor of Biochemistry spoke harshly to us when we backed into his car. It is exceedingly cold, and Ernie is on holiday.

Outpost of Empire

SINCE our translation to an outpost of Empire we have become steadily more sophisticated, and nothing much surprises us any more. True, we have not yet ceased to react pleasurably at the sight of a flock of green parrots sitting on the roof of the Physiology department, and the undoubted presence of scorpions in the sand outside Anatomy still induces a delightful gooseflesh in our sandalled feet. But when a ghastly tumult breaks out over our heads in the middle of a tutorial we no

longer turn pale and falter, for we recognise the characteristic
sound of possums pursued by the animal-house cat. We have
grown accustomed to lecturing to dogs of all shapes and sizes,
sometimes curled up in the one and ninepennies, and sometimes crouched under the lecturer's bench, ready to spring. The
other day one of them—a black-and-white spotted affair—got up
in the middle of our lecture, yawned widely, and stalked out.
We did not even blink.

Nevertheless our new community lecture theatre has given
us pause. The room doubles as a Histology laboratory, and is
therefore long and flat, in contrast to the precipitous cliffside we
were wont to confront. Indeed, it is only on exceptionally clear
days that we can see the back bench from the dais. The roof is
low and the temperature high, a circumstance dictating the
opening of windows which admit the full roar of the heavy
traffic and the happy screams of the patrons of the bathing
beach outside. We have all become hoarse in the attempt to
transfer the cargo of our overburdened minds to the keeping of
our young friends in the back row, but our biochemist has
finally cracked under the strain, and we are waiting for a public
address system which will allow us to harangue the multitude
at the cost of fewer petechial haemorrhages. In the meantime
our electrophysiologist has kindly rigged us up an imposing
assembly of apparatus which subserves roughly the same purpose. We have a rickety microphone which we clutch feverishly
to our teeth, and our thoughts pass through two black metallic
boxes under the bench to a loud-speaker placed on the floor
close to the door—an object of keen scrutiny from our canine
visitors.

In the first box, as in all electronic apparatus we have met,
there is a bewildering array of knobs, in this case freely labelled
with slogans like 'Bass up', 'Record', or 'Tone', which we take
to be Hi-Fi stigmata. If we injudiciously leave the microphone to
its own devices while we write on the blackboard, it yells and
howls till we get back to it again and can twiddle one of the
knobs to calm it. We are not very good at electrons, but our electrophysiologist has given us a thorough coaching on which
knob to turn. For a time all went well, but our undoing came
yesterday, when in the heat of one of our impassioned per-
orations we arrogantly turned a knob without bending down to
make the vital identification. Instantly the loudspeaker began

to pour forth a stream of abstruse biochemical information, delivered in the voice of our ingenious biochemist and amplified to several thousand decibels.

It was not until morning tea that we stopped twitching sufficiently for it to be explained to us slowly and carefully that the *second* black box contained a tape-recorder.

Committee Man

THERE was a time (it seems odd to think of it now) when we knew very little about libraries. We began our official career as a custodian of books some years ago, as a member of the Preclinical Library Committee, recommending books in a carefree way and adopting a proprietorial air over the journal racks when we visited our domain. By diligent attention to detail we rapidly climbed the ladder of promotion to the post of Chairman, and in counsel with our studious and reliable Preclinical Librarian we developed such striking lines of policy as the provision of red linoleum for the floor and the planting of flame-trees outside the windows to keep the sun off. We even asked the university for an air-conditioning unit so that the students might read without the risk of heat exhaustion. Naturally, subversive notions of this kind could not be tolerated in any respectable university, and we awoke one morning to find that we had been kicked upstairs into membership of the University Library Committee itself. This body operates on an altogether more rarefied plane, meeting in the Vice-Chancellor's room and fortifying itself with tea and chocolate biscuits.

After our translation we made a general tour of the University Library to examine the ramifications of our new responsibility. We prowled at will through the forbidden hinterland, entering the reference staff-room, the cataloguing staff-room, the orders room, and the acquisitions department. We visited the bindery, the photographic room, and the book-lift. A chat on logistics with our learned and genial Librarian revealed to us that each undergraduate reader required 25 sq. ft. of space, and each postgraduate 35 sq. ft., that the accepted ratio of seats to full-time students is 1:3, and that the standard height of book stacks is 7 ft. 6 in. The whole atmosphere was quiet and scholarly, far removed from that of our early struggles in the Preclinical Library.

Finally we visited the reading-rooms. The books did not frighten us so much—after all, we had been nipping in and out to borrow Trollope for years, and it had not escaped our notice that there were other sorts of books around—it was the journals which pointed up our narrow-minded professional outlook. In agriculture, for example, it seems that they read *Beef Situation* and *Herbage Abstracts*. The chemists receive, among others, the *Perfumery and Essential Oil Record*, and *Pipe Roll Society* is required reading for lawyers. In education they spend happy hours reading *Let's Dance*, or, more soberly, *Laban Art of Movement*, and, for a dreamy mood, the enigmatic *Etude*. The zoologists are addicted to *Insects Sociaux* and *Tuatara*, and the psychologists find instruction as well as relaxation in studying the *Journal of Projective Technique*. The engineers—solid earthy creatures— while away their long weekends with *Beama, Diesel Engine Users' Association*, and *Muck Shifter*.

At the next meeting of the Library Committee I am going to suggest that some of these journals should be routed through the Preclinical Library to broaden, for the medical student, the straitened educational experience which we all so much deplore. It is safe to say that no-one could read *Muck Shifter* and remain unbroadened, and a study of *Beef Situation* could only expand the restricted technical horizon. In return we could offer the Faculty of Arts a choice of *Brain* or *Gut*, and the Faculty of Education might like to glance through a few recent issues of *Blood*.

Tin Tray

THE ordering system in our department is complex, with numerous highly coloured forms to be signed in triplicate. Just recently it became our duty to sign them, and we were fascinated to find what the department had been running on all these years. We even got round to making tentative little inquiries of our formidable senior technician when we found him in a good mood. 'What,' we would ask timidly, 'do we *do* with all these assorted grummets?'

After a time we became a little bolder and actually attempted to strike out one or two items, but it made no difference; they always came back on the next order form, and we were given to understand that interference of this sort made the department almost impossible to run. Eventually we became almost anaesthetic, and nowadays we sign our name without a moment's thought to '36 only alum. pudd. steamers, complete with lid'.

But the other day our eye was caught by an item reading:

> '1 only tin tray with picture ..   .. 4s. 0d.'

We no longer dare to approach our senior technician on matters of this kind, but we sent at once for our new secretary, who is always glad to enlighten us. It seems that the Professor's tea tray had become a Disgrace, that a tin tray with a picture on it is cheaper than a tin tray without one, and that the picture would almost certainly prove to be a spaniel, the trade considering spaniels to have maximum sales appeal.

Convinced by these telling arguments, we signed without demur, and it was not until the matter came up at the afternoon tea club yesterday that we remembered that the Professor is greatly attached to his fox-terrier. A rough canvass of departmental opinion only too clearly supported our fear that the appearance of a spaniel might be regarded as a studied insult. It was widely felt that we had been too precipitate, and should have specified a psychologically neutral picture. We were forced to speak sharply to one of our demonstrators, and our senior lecturer, who owns a Siamese cat, referred slightingly to dogs in general. At this a visiting dog-lover from Biochemistry swallowed a cigarette in his agitation, and had to be revived with copious draughts of hot water. The meeting broke up in a general huff, and our migraine came on worse than ever.

It was therefore with some relief that we welcomed this morning an end to the suspense in the shape of the arrival of the tray itself. 'We have pleasure' said the accompanying letter suavely, 'in supplying to your specificaion 1 only tin tray with picture, price 4s. 0d., and trust that it will meet your requirements adequately.' With trembling fingers we undid the string. It was, of course, *The Boyhood of Raleigh*.

Before Xerox

IN our department we are a conservative lot. The strain of maintaining our fevered thought-processes in working order leaves us little time for consideration of our material surroundings, and we are well behind the times. The Professor's dictaphone has valves instead of transistors, and we haven't an electric typewriter in the place. But creakingly and slowly we progress. Take the duplicator, for instance. Our duplicator dates from well before there is any record of Man in the department, and since we were so high we have been accustomed to see it sulking in the corner of the practical classroom. On feast days it is run out by a team of our indefatigable secretaries fully attired in anti-duplicator clothing, and after a series of propitiatory rites it begins clankingly to duplicate. Some four hours later, when three stencils have been ruined and several reams of paper spoiled, we have a hundred copies of our terminal examination paper to distribute to the unappreciative multitude. Our disillusioned cleaners then undertake the mopping-up operations, and the duplicator team spends the rest of the day sitting round a winchester of ether—they have used three this year already—removing the ink from their persons.

Such is the standard procedure, the norm of duplication. Most of us would not have it otherwise. But there is a radical undertow in the department, and last Tuesday the chap came to demonstrate a new duplicator. It was a solemn moment. A hushed semicircle assembled in the classroom, and the machine was reverently led in, mounted on noiseless white-wall tyres and attended cautiously by the Professor's dog. It had everything. It would duplicate in sixteen different colours; it would reproduce wiring diagrams and pictures of the west front of Wells Cathedral; it was filled through a service port by means of an enormous toothpaste tube without a drop of the ink becoming visible on its exterior; it had in its bowels a reserve tank swinging on gimbals; it had a tinsel brush to discourage static. A small tray pulled out to hold coffee cups, and in the elegant substructure there was a compartment for cake. You simply switch it on, the chap said, and when it has finished it rings a bell and shuts itself off. At this the Professor's dog howled mournfully, but to no avail; the committee was already sold, hypnotised by the thought of Christmas cards in sixteen colours and the possibility of the machine doubling as a coffee bar on Saturdays. The model we have been allotted is obviously eager to start. The day it came the bell rang continuously for seven minutes and the machine edged its way into the centre of the room, where it hummed industriously for some time before shutting itself off with an expectant quiver. We are determined it shall not feel it is wasting its talents with us, and we are giving the students an extra examination at the beginning of term so that it shall not consider itself neglected.

Intercom

IT is becoming increasingly clear that the audio-visual aids in our department are hopelessly out of date. We have no fluorescent chalk for passing messages to our staff during a blacked-out conference, nor do our specimens glow softly in the dark when we lecture to the students. We have no multiple stethoscope, no remote-controlled projector. The years slip by and we haven't made one teaching film. When we looked at our stereoscope the other day a big fat spider ran out. We haven't even had two-way television installed. But worst of all is our communications system. We remember being terribly impressed when we visited a teaching hospital recently and timidly enquired for an acquaintance of ours. Within ten seconds the corridors were reverberating to the summons we had initiated. 'Calling Dr. Kildare!' the loudspeakers said—just like the movies. It is true that our acquaintance was eventually located in his room, where a simple telephone call would have sufficed to find him, but the general electronic effect was most impressive. How different from our own intercom!

When a major crisis develops and we must have help immediately we simply tell the lab. boy to nip down and ask if tea is up yet. There are no buzzers, no red and green flashing lights, no electrons. When we come to think of it, we are still using the system the ancient Egyptians must have used. Not long ago we read that the patients in some hospitals are to be fitted out with telephones, and in desperation our colleagues have been

practising against the great day when we too will have adequate
liaison between one part of our department and another. 'Hello
three, hello three!' they call out of the window, 'Come and get
it, repeat get it! Out!' And from the storey above there comes
a faint bellow 'Hello two, hello two! Roger! Out!'

Sterilizer

WE have a steriliser in the passage outside our lab. to deal with
the animal-house cages. In the old days it was a large cubical
galvanised box in which steam was generated by the judicious
insertion of electrons and water, and a child could see how it
worked. Indeed, after a few hours of operation other senses
than sight came into play, and most of us could nominate the
species from which the contents had been derived. Meanwhile
steam leaked gently from every available point, and the temperature of the whole building rose steadily to heat exhaustion
level. To adapt a legal phrase, not only was sterilisation done,
it also manifestly appeared to be done.

We have, however, changed all that. The new steriliser arrived
the other day and is now finally installed. It is an imposing
cylindrical structure, crouched in a corner in a veil of gaily
painted pipes. There are dials to tell us when it is about to
explode, and by opening some of the fourteen taps and closing
others it is possible to bundle parcels of steam from point to
point in the interior. There are oil-immersion switches, mercury
contact-breakers, rheostats, and a clock by which we all set out
watches. Now then, we said, no more sodden notebooks, no
more rusty typewriters.

Alas, we have but exchanged our whips for scorpions. In
the bowels of the machine there is what we understand to
be a solenoid which opens and shuts something with a reverberating and irregular clang of such penetrative power that it
has already caused cups of tea to be spilled in adjacent departments and a visiting R.A.F. type to become airborne. Plaster is
falling steadily throughout the building, and ominous cracks
have appeared in the outside wall. Moreover, while the effects
of opening certain taps are on balance beneficial, opening others
causes vast quantities of superheated steam from the 20th
century to disappear into the plumbing system inadequate for

the demands of the 19th, with an unearthly rushing sound. Windows rattle, test-tubes tilt and shatter, and learned conversation breaks up into a string of oaths.

For our part, the animals can take their chance: what we always say is, soap and water were good enough for us.

Projector Assembly

OUR new projector arrived the other day, in a couple of imposing packing-cases, and we all assembled eagerly on the chance of being allowed to play with it. The *Instruction and Service Manual* began in a restrained motherly key:

'Unscrew the lid of the large case and lift out the cabinet, taking care not to scratch the finish . . . clean out the inside of the cabinet and dust the screen carefully . . . gently lift it from the case and remove the cross batten . . . make sure you have thoroughly washed behind the ears.'

For the next two pages all was sweetness and light; a paragraph was devoted to the discovery of the main switch A, and another to the identification of the earth wire marked *Earth*. A fleeting chill ran down our spines over two sinister nuts T1 and T2 which had to be exactly $7^{29}/_{32}$ in. (19.97 cm.) apart; but otherwise the gentle flow of Instruction soothed and relaxed us. It was just like 'Meccano'.

This could not last, and by the fourth page a peevish admonitory note had crept in: 'Ensure that the shutter-operating pin P, if removed, is replaced square end up.' This began the rot. Search as we might, we could discover no trace of the shutter-operating pin P, or indeed of its square end. We could locate the coupling screw K, the counter-balance arm R, the operating cams and slide claw, and for that matter the locking nut Y and the spring and collar Q. But no shutter-operating pin P.

At this point we discovered that the milled knobs G looked vaguely unfamiliar, and that there was no sign of the hand-control knob E or the pair of knurled screws H. We are scientists—men trained to assess evidence. A glance at fig. 7 confirmed that we had spent an hour assembling one type of instrument with the manual intended for another. Our professor is even more scientific; when the matter was brought before him, it took him only half an hour to discover that he had ordered and received an instrument not designed for projecting at all.

Innumeracy

A friend of ours who proudly possesses a rather exotic thermocouple buttonholed us the other day. It seems he was approached by a psychologically minded colleague whose ambition it was to record the thermal changes engendered in his skin by psychological traumata. Our friend was delighted to demonstrate his electronic skill, but was momentarily taken aback to find that he was expected also to supply the psychological traumata. 'What do you expect me to do?' he asked doubtfully. 'Oh, just insult me,' said the psychologist, stirring impatiently in his chair, 'anything will do.' Opportunities of this sort are rare enough in the Welfare State, and our friend was somewhat out of practice. He essayed a few tentative remarks on his visitor's physical appearance and dress; the psychologist smiled blandly. Warming to his task, he cast aspersions on the psychologist's ancestry and relations; the psychologist crossed his legs and examined the ceiling. Finally our friend animadverted on the intimate habits and moral short-comings of his guest; the skin-temperature went down half a degree and the psychologist stifled a yawn. Our friend retreated, baffled, and put the case to the lab. man outside, an embittered and disillusioned character of great resource. 'Ask him to add up a sum,' said the lab man, 'no psychologist knows any arithmetic.' Our friend returned to battle, and found the psychologist examining the thermocouple with ill-disguised contempt. 'What are seventeen seventeens?' he demanded fiercely, 'quick, now!' A slow flush mounted to the psychologist's cheeks and his lips trembled. 'Seventeen seven-teens' he repeated weakly, 'let me see, let me see.' The needle trembled and shot up; the day was won. Five minutes later the psychologist had called for pen and paper, and finally crept out, a beaten man. Our friend understands that his thermocouple will not be needed after all.

Conditions de vente

HAVING recently had occasion to inquire into the possibility of purchasing some electrical apparatus, we found ourselves led insensibly into a series of communications with an old-established French firm. Our latest receipt in this correspondence is a schedule entitled *Conditions de vente*, which appears to contain the nub or crux of the projected transaction. It is a complicated document, and after several pages concerned with such matters as *expedition*, *délai*, etc., we came at last to the vital factor of *prix*. This factor proved unexpectedly difficult to elucidate, being surrounded by a scientific smoke-screen of Gallic exuberance and plasticity. The section began forbiddingly:

'*Nos prix sont révisables suivant la formule*

$$P = P_o \left(0,10 + 0,80 \frac{S}{S_o} + 0,10 \frac{M}{M_o} \right)$$

où les différents paramètres sont définis ainsi: – . . . '

But we are made of stern stuff, undaunted by income-tax schedules and claims for mileage allowance; dragging to our bosom our invaluable New Little Larousse, we ploughed on. It appeared that P was the definitive price, P_o the estimated price, S the index of wages in the Electrical and related industries published (and rectified globally) by a mysterious body designated R.G.E. two months before the actual date of delivery, and S_o the index for the fortnight preceding the date of the estimate. M_o was the price of aluminium in sheets of 1 mm. (R.G.E.), and M the value on the last day of the first two-thirds of the actual delay in delivery. When we had got thus far our attention was distracted by a musical plash, and we observed with interest that a drop of sweat from our overheated brow had fallen on the paper. All we had wanted originally was a galvanometer, but we no longer felt the desire.

On the other hand, when we showed the document to one of our clinical colleagues who is still fortunate enough to have a few private patients he was at once interested, and he has produced a sliding scale of fees based on a similar principle. His

final charge (F) is related to the estimate given to the patient (E)
by the following equation:

$$F = E \left(0.1 + 0.5 \frac{C}{C_0} + 0.2 \frac{P}{P_0} + 0.2 \frac{T}{T_0} \right)^n + \sqrt{D_c, D_w}$$

where C is the mean cost-of-living index in the period between
the operation and the rendering of the account, and C_0 the index
figure at the time of arranging admission. P and P_0 represent
the corresponding figures for the cost of petrol, and T and T_0
those for telephone rental. D_c and D_w represent physical depre-
ciation of our colleague and his wife in units of earning and
coping capacity respectively, and the exponential n has been
added by a statistical friend who feels vaguely uneasy without it.

Safe Breaker

ONE of our colleagues is an inoffensive man we knew as a
physiologist, but who is now Working for the Ministry. His
metamorphosis involved the security screening of everyone
inside the department and almost everyone outside it. It also
involved a safe. The safe was a combination model, opened
with a key and a word of four letters, and our colleague watched
it arrive from the makers complete with key but less the combination, which was to arrive the next day by Safe Hand. All
the lawless instincts of a *ci-devant* physiologist stirred to life.
He fetched a stethoscope to listen to the tumblers, limbered up
his fingers, and set to work.

His first attempt was to try all the rude words which could be
formed from an implausible collection of consonants. While
thus engaged he happened to turn one knob briskly in an anti-
clockwise direction and it came away in his hand, leaving a
small hexagonal hole leading into the bowels of the safe. Ten
minutes later, when there were four hexagonal holes leading
into the bowels of the safe, our colleague suddenly realised that
each knob could be reinserted in six different positions in each
of four different holes and that he had omitted to take notes.
Hastily replacing the knobs at random, he retired to establish an
alibi, having carefully wiped the safe and knobs to remove
fingerprints.

His interview with the Safe Hand the next day defies transcription, but it ended in the engineer from Birmingham being sent for. It took him two days.

Electron Suppression

A PRECLINICAL colleague of ours has a profound distrust of electrons, even when suitably emboxed and under the strict surveillance of an expert. It appears that this distrust is mutual, for he has always been able to exert an inimical influence on the performance of any electrical apparatus merely by his presence in the vicinity. At his approach his friends cover up their electric clocks and muffle their refrigerators. In his lab. they have learned by experience to keep the thermostats in the basement and the embedding ovens in inaccessible corners.

Judge then of our colleague's dismay on finding that in his absence abroad his room had become the seat of feverish electrical activity. The whole of one bench was submerged beneath a smothering blanket of condensers, amplifiers and rectifiers, while there were also several sinister black japanned cases mounted on rubber and undoubtedly containing numerous valves of the small malignant kind which never fit into any socket. Beneath the bench lurked two enormous batteries, and in the window, on his favourite seat, there stood the final ignominy, a trickle-charger. The floor was knee-deep in wire.

Our friend at once recognised the spoor of the electrophysiologist next door, who had not expected him back so soon. His wrath rose, and he said a naughty word. Revenge, however, was easy. He walked slowly round the room, pausing before each individual component of the prevailing chaos and fixing it solemnly with his eye. The immediate results were not spectacular, but the long-range effects are mounting daily. The apparatus has to all appearances been safely removed, but our colleague understands that square-wave pulses have been replaced by monophasic spikes, that the trickle-charger has caused acid to splutter all over various electrophysiological objets d'art, and that several dollar-consuming valves have blown. He is confident there will be no further encroachments the next time he goes abroad.

The Masterpiece

IT is now some time since we became tired of writing scientific papers in which nobody was interested. We felt that our psyche was cramped by these endless processions of *facts*, the limitless calvacade of introductions, techniques, results, discussions, and summaries, with their subsidiary acknowledgements, references, and illustrations. It came to us that what we needed was an outlet for our personality, a larger canvas for our brush. We determined to let our soul take wings. We would write a book.

Initially we detected a pervading apathy among the various publishers we attempted to favour with our custom. 'We recognise, of course,' their letters began, 'that the work you have been doing is of first-rate importance, but . . . ' Eventually, however, we succeeded in discovering a kindly firm who were sorry for us, and obtained an imposing-looking memorandum covered in red seals, in which we were hereinafter described as the author.

The first proofs arrived heavily annotated in a fine Italianate script by the translator. 'Cytoarchitectonics of the Umbilicus', we had written baldly, '1. The Philosophical Background.' This had now become Perp. Titl. 258 12 pt. cap. # d. 1½ pts. R4 rule 24 ems. Sub. Perp. 239 18 pt. fig. ital. caps. No. ⊙ s', and we were delighted to find ourselves so much in the technical swim. We discoursed at length to our colleagues at morning tea on the relative advantages of Times bold face and Garamond in the production of scientific literature, and at lunchtime we went out and bought a spotted bow tie. In the afternoon, however, we were mildly dashed to find, lurking among the pages, little interdepartmental publisher's messages. They began innocently enough with 'Margin sheet pl.', but soon we began to detect a somewhat censorious hectoring attitude. 'Charlie,' read the second, 'doubtful Latin p. 15.' Others were briefer, but not less to the point. 'C.P.', they said, marking our favourite purple passage, '? constr. Yrs. E.R.' After a time relations between C.P. and E.R. became slightly strained, and a brisk argument developed (over our prostrate body) on a grammatical point on p.127. But on the whole we saw no cause for serious alarm, and we relaxed into a happy daze of authorship.

Our first intimation that all was not well came with the arrival of the first press copies, in a parcel bearing the bold-face label OF NO COMMERCIAL VALUE. Since then we have seen all too clearly what they meant. The reviewers have on the whole been tolerant, but they have made it clear that this has been a difficult task. 'Too long', they said, stifling a yawn. 'Too short', said others impatiently. 'Too detailed', said the clinical types, throwing down their pens to dash off to a subtotal viscerectomy. 'Too vague', said the back-room boys with scarcely concealed contempt. 'Too orthodox; too speculative; too turgid; too simple; unsuitable for students, unsuitable for teachers, unsuitable for research workers, unsuitable . . . '

The other day a distinguished guest was rummaging about in our library of *Penguins* when we heard our youngest child say to him in a sad meditative voice, 'My Daddy wrote a book once. It didn't sell.'

Scientific Books

SOME years ago I was rash enough to buy a book. I forget what it was—something to do with first-aid, probably, or the care and maintenance of the golden hamster. Anyway, I asked them to charge it, and from that moment dates my inferiority complex. They have got it into their heads that I am a good prospect, an easy touch, and not a week passes but they send me a catalogue of *New and Forthcoming Scientific Books*. Every fourth or fifth week I receive a catalogue (slightly foxed) of *Old and Rare Scientific Books*, and every two or three months—so bewildering is our English climate—there arrives the *Autumn List of Scientific Books*.

It is these catalogues that depress me, particularly the mathematical section. These chaps don't fiddle around with experiments. They *know*. It is impossible to read the brief chapter headings without a stirring of the emotions. The Hopf Invariant; Fibre Spaces; the Hurewicz Theorems; how they would reverberate in the mind of the reader! Or again, Some Fundamental Properties of Noetherian Rings; Residue Rings and Rings of Quotients; A New List of P-multiplied Laplace Transforms; these are the very stuff of science, the life's blood of the future.

When I have read through the catalogues I often go along to the animal house and look at all those rabbits and feel quite low in my mind. Last week I felt so badly about it I went out and bought another book.

The Library Revisited

NOW that I am retired I naturally have to spend most of my time looking for my spectacles, trying to remember the names of my grandchildren, and wondering what I meant to do when I opened the cupboard door just now. But at intervals I manage to wander along to the medical library to see how far they have gone to the dogs without my regular partronage.

I first frequented medical libraries in the golden era when they were peaceful temples of helpful information; the annual input to the *Index Medicus* was contained in a single manageable volume, and symposia had not yet begun to breed. I was allowed by silver-haired librarians to sit in a comfortable chair in a dimly lit corner and occupy myself with a few slim books or journals. Clocks ticked, dust motes floated, and an occasional cough merely drew attention to the blissful silence.

Nowadays things are different. The present librarian has not a single silver hair (librarians, like policemen, grow younger every year). The stacks are in a constant state of flux, so that nothing is where it was last time, and every desirable current journal is either at the binders or has been stolen. The construction of the plastic seats bears no vestige of relationship to the construction of the bodies they are supposed to support, and the strip lights dazzle the eyes of the reader. Borrowing a book has become an electronic intelligence test which I cannot pass, and there is constant noise pollution from slot-machine copiers. In all directions lurk the cold glares of visual display units; Big Brother is still watching us, even though it is now 1985.

But these are minor hazards; it is the printed page itself that distresses me most. Once upon a time readers sat down to articles like 'On the comparative structure of the cortex cerebri', or 'Traité de la venin de la vipère; on y a joint un description d'un nouveau canal de l'oeil', in the confident expectation of enjoying a rattling good yarn. Today even the lists of contents of most of the journals are incomprehensible because of esoteric chemical formulae, arcane hormonal axes, and mysterious immunological or genetic jargon; I never dare to look inside. Nor do the Recent Acquisitions cheer me up; these 800-page monsters merely reinforce my resentment that so many people know so much about things of which I am entirely ignorant.

However, I am glad to say that I can still (usually) understand every word in *In England Now*, and this enables me to return home somewhat comforted.

Franking Letters

ONCE upon a time we were connected with an International Congress, and since then nothing in our correspondence surprises us any more. We are, in fact, just about the most blasé correspondent we know. There was a time when the blunt word 'Drukwerk' on the front of a postcard would send the blood coursing wildly through our arteriovenous anastomoses, and we even used to attempt to translate the body of the communication. Nowadays we simply reach out for a reprint—*any* reprint— and send it off madly in all directions. 'Brevkort', Briefkaart', 'Impresos'—they are all the same to us, and even 'Matbua' arouses in us only a sluggish momentary question. We might as well admit that we are completely foxed by the piece that begins 'Bizi çok ilgilendiren aşağidaki çalişmalariniz-dan . . . ', and our Hungarian is not what it might be. Our lack of enthusiasm extends to the outside of our missives as well. Our eyes slide unheedingly over the slogans on the outside of the envelope. 'Post early for Christmas!' is the anxious cry of the feckless British; 'Indiquez votre nom et votre adresse au verso de vos lettres' say our prudent neighbours suavely; while the industrial motif comes to the top with such offerings as 'Frankfurt A.M., Zentrum des internationalen Verkehrs.' 'K.V.N.Ø.F.S.o.s.v.' exhort the Danes mysteriously; 'Secours Suisse d'hiver' remind the Swiss. But the Americans are better at this sort of thing than any European. They are not hampered by sober industrious inhibitions. The other day we got a large gaily coloured card franked with the legend 'Evolution is Bunk!'—a claim at once plausible, educative, and interesting.

And only this morning our attention was momentarily diverted by a large and ferocious Indian in full war-paint—outlined, appropriately enough, in red ink—on the front of a letter from a colleague in Florida. By the side of this impressive figure is the blood-curdling conjuration—'Scalp 'em, Seminoles!'

Fan Mail

I have always been impressed by the extent and variety of my colleagues' fan mail. From all quarters of the free and occupied globe the letters pour in, and the postcards requesting reprints are neatly stacked in their rooms according to the country of origin. A brisk trade in stamps is done, and their children are well up in the latest Peruvian and Senegalese issues. No sooner does one of my acquaintances express himself in print than the obsequious missives begin. 'Illustrious and honoured Professor,' they write cringingly to our new junior research assistant, 'the world is richer for your work. Will you please have the gratitude to send me ten copies. Accept, I pray, my compliments the most distinguished. I remain, illustrious Professor, Scribble-Scratch, Over-Chief of Clinic.'

My own publications arouse minimal enthusiasm, and I never have any stamps to swap. Occasionally at the end of a long and scurrilous letter on other subjects there occurs some such phrase as 'Your last effort wasn't such tripe as usual—send us along a reprint, will you?'; but there is no emotion, no soul, in such requests. It is true that I once received an indecipherable postcard from Hungary, and on one glorious morning a letter arrived for me from Guam; I let it lie for a day to sink into my colleagues' subconscious. Alas, it proved to be a request for an article written by a namesake of mine in a rival establishment.

If this were all it would not be so bad. But the other requests that arrive are equally humiliating. My friends spend their time attending conferences in Rio or congresses in Brno—always by invitation, and usually to open the proceedings—and keep their hands in during the close season by dropping into the Royal Society to read one or two papers. In the winter evenings they are asked to talk on the Third Programme or they dash off a book at the humble request of the publishers.

My own life is very different. My books are always sent to cynical readers who return them with such comments as 'Style pedestrian; content uncritical; limited public only.' If I attend a congress it is always in Birmingham, and my paper is always taken as read because the time-table has fallen into desuetude. But I have had my moment. The other day a colleague travelled sixty miles on the British Railways accompanied by a decapitated head of a ferret in a paper bag to ask me what in my opinion were the names of the muscles in its neck.

Professors

IN the comics, there are only two kinds of professor. One is the scientist whose mind has become overheated and warped, so that he is planning to use the cosmic rays to blast the earth to the neighbourhood of Proxima Centauri, where his masters, the gigantic slug-like creatures who control the Galactic Federation, can take over. The other is the professor who has become divorced from reality by too much study, so that he continually allows himself to be captured by international spies. Even when rescued by the Fifth Form Gang at St. Christopher's he is a liability, and has to be led about and fed, because he can't even remember to eat. Both kinds of professor wear beards; the first a short thick black affair to conceal his weak chin and cruel mouth, and the second a long grey straggling one which is usually thickly encrusted with egg.

Brought up on material of this kind, the adult lay population regards real life professors as unreliable and unbalanced creatures. Nevertheless, science and medical professors who achieve the ultimate in success by having a potted version of their work published in the Reader's Digest are at once pigeon-holed by the communications industry as geniuses—until they start the cosmic ray business, that is—and their utterances on any subject become infallible. No sooner does a professor discover something—perhaps a new pathway for the break-down of an obscure peptide in the liver of the greater spotted woodpecker—than the Sunday press features in detail his views on marriage guidance, the current situation in Roumania, and

Mr. Arthur Scargill. Professors who make no discoveries are not considered a social asset and are not asked their views. Nor are they asked to sherry parties or to appear on television quiz programmes.

University administrators regard medical professors as obstructive individualists whose sole aim is to sabotage the orderly running of the institution. There are the prima donnas, who stamp in to resign because the office has knocked back their request for a strip light over the new research assistant's coffee pot. There are the secret agents, who never fill in proformas, and conceal the details of their courses so successfully that nobody is sure how many students they have and what they are doing with them. There are the Public Figures, who spell out the inefficiency of the administration on television, and there are the sullen introverts who refuse to be put on committees or to be civil to the chap who organizes the timetable. The administrative view of professors is thus that they are potentially dangerous psychopaths.

In fact, nearly everyone, even including many professors, thinks that professors are mad. It is certainly true that if they are not mad when they take office, they have every reason for rapidly becoming so. There are the daily worries, such as the question of raising the subscription to the tea club, tracking down a missing library book, or calming a visiting research fellow who has nowhere to park his car. The longer term problems include planning the new department which all professors expect will at any moment take the place of the present ridiculously cramped accommodation. Some of the more gullible ones spend years in detailed architectural study, drawing up one plan after another, before it dawns on them that they are not going to get a new department after all.

Most toxic of all are the meetings, to which professors are nowadays expected to devote something like three-quarters of their time. If a professor, more foolhardy than the rest, decides not to go to one of these interminable sessions he is subsequently informed that, because he wasn't there to defend himself, he has been appointed to the committee planning the fifth or sixth new curriculum in the last five years. Every vacation is the signal for an intensification of the showers of agenda and minutes, for the administration thinks that once the students have dispersed to the ski slopes or the beaches the professors may get bored from lack of occupation. (This is directly traceable to the comics the administrators read in their early youth.) Also in the vacations come the piles of examination scripts, the incomprehensible and unworkable timetables for next year, the research grant reports, the estimation of the departmental expenditure and the checking of the departmental inventory. It is small wonder that during the deliberations of the curriculum committee the weaker and more frail professors may be found dozing, and have to be rapped sharply on the head with a ruler by the Faculty Secretary.

Nowadays lectures are out of fashion, and ever more complex systems of teaching are continually being devised. Seminars, symposia, workshops, conferences, debates, and so on, all require three to four times as much preparation as a straight-forward lecture, usually lead to bad feeling among the staff concerned, and are often regarded by the students as third-rate music-hall entertainment.

External examining can be a diversion from such experiences, but it is a two-edged diversion. The bad side of it includes marking the papers and the fact that the external examiner is always allotted the borderline students, so that when it comes to the orals no interesting questions can be asked, and it can be very dull. On the other hand there are occasional bonuses, as when a young lady was handed a temporal bone by the examiner and asked, by way of opening the conversation with an easy one: 'How many of these do you have?' After some calculation she said 'Five'. 'Five!' said the examiner, 'how do you make that out?' 'Well', she said, 'I have two in my head and one in my hand, and I'm four months pregnant.'

When the professor returns from one of these expeditions he usually finds that all the sessions of the committees on which he sits are not, as he innocently imagined, safely over and done with, but have been postponed till his return since his presence was felt to be essential.

In the odd chinks of time between the end of one of these meetings and the hour at which the whistle blows for the next, the professor may drag his weary mind into his laboratory, where the spiders disport themselves among his rusting apparatus. Here he turns for a few brief moments to the contemplation of what in his youth he fondly thought was to be his life work. He is at once in trouble. In his carefree days as a

Senior Lecturer he could cite you a reference as well as the next
man, and set up as neat an experiment as anyone could wish.
Ideas fermented in his skull to burst forth later into print. But
now, when he sits down in front of his bench, what can he
remember? Usually nothing except the decision of the Senatus
to appoint a subcommittee to investigate the possibility of setting up a working party which would report to the standing
committee on staff/student ratios in the Faculty of Arts on the
proposals contained in a memorandum at a conference which
everyone has now forgotten. It is not surprising that so few professors are Fellows of the Royal Society.

Taking everything into consideration, the definition which I
would apply to most professors is the one that Dr. Johnson
applied to himself in the great dictionary which he compiled. A
lexicographer, according to Dr. Johnson, is a 'harmless drudge',
and this is as good a description of a professor as any.

Dressage and Diet

ON a recent visit to the dentist a dietician friend of ours looked
round the waiting room for reading matter which might distract
her from contemplation of the forthcoming session. The only
thing currently available was a journal devoted to horses, with
a natural penumbra of equipment, eventing, dressage, hacking
and racing. It was scarcely the sort of distraction our friend had
in mind, but any port in a storm.

She began with an advertisement: 'This Christmas, say "I
love you" with a saddle', an idea which would certainly not
have occurred spontaneously to our friend. Greatly encouraged,
she embarked on an article on the Half Halt, which, she learned,
must on no account be confused with the Incomplete Halt, and
is called the Parade in France. 'If you can't apply a parade',
asked the journal querulously, 'how can you really influence the
horse? How can you engage him, create impulsion, elevate his
forehand, influence him to work with lightness and gaiety?'

This rhetoric was too deep for our friend, and she passed to
the next advertisement, which, by a happy chance, appeared to
solve the problem for those unable to apply a parade. 'Horse
Mixes', it stressed, 'are not just a dietary supplement, they

improve appetite, balance the pH in the digestive system, raise the blood count more rapidly, dramatically change condition and appearance, and improve breeding performance.'

Our friend's professional instincts were at once aroused, and as she read she became convinced that Horse Mixes might easily engage, and create impulsion in, some of her intractable patients, whose condition and appearance badly needed changing; they might even be influenced to work with lightness and gaiety, though this was less likely. She had doubts about elevating their forehands, and felt rather diffident about assessing possible improvements in their breeding performance. At all events she intends to explore the matter fully, and has sent away for the Free Explanatory Booklet in full colour.

Animal Catalogue

YOU can see we are a dull lot in our department if you come and look at our animal-house. There are a few mice, a number of sinister-looking variegated rabbits, and an altogether excessive accumulation of plain white rats. No tropical fish, no snakes, no piglets. In other departments one can entertain visiting firemen for hours merely by taking them to see the baboons or the porcupines, but the entertainment rating of our animal-house is nil.

The whole thing is a great trial to our patient and industrious administrator. In spite of a number of years spent in tracking down mysterious leaks of D.C. current, distributing cleaning materials, cataloguing the Professor's library, and reprimanding the recalcitrant students, she retains an incurably romantic disposition in respect of this matter of animals. When we called on her the other day to ask about our dirty windows we found her just finishing a telephone conversation. 'Well,' she was saying, 'if you don't know when the frogs are going to come in, could you at least put me on the waiting-list for salamanders?' She put down the telephone and showed us a catalogue she had received that morning. 'Why don't you try something different?' she asked and we thought we could detect an incipient curl of the lip. It was indeed a stirring catalogue. We reluctantly rejected the Elephants (each £750 F.O.B. Singapore),

the Tigers (each £325 – £350), and the Black Panthers (£325), all
in Splendid Health and Condition and our eye wandered down
through the Slow Lories, the Binturongs, and the Ursine Tree
Kangaroos (each £40) to the Black Headed Munia and the Green
White Eye Brows (each 10s.). We considered a pair of Redrumps
at £5 or a pair of Twentyeights at £14.10s., and noted with
interest that the prices of Lions, Giraffes, Zebras, Hippopotami,
and Shetland Ponies were all subject to market fluctuations.
Finally we settled for a couple of Turtles for Aquariums
(small)—each 5s.

But we fear that our enterprising order has done little to
improve matters. As we left, the phone rang again. It was Pathology, wanting to borrow some mice. Our administrator was
quite sharp with them.

Beaver Dam

A colleague of ours in the States whose interests run to comparative physiology told us of a harassing experience. It appears
that our colleague became interested in the matter of beavers,
but was unfortunate enough to live in a virtually beaverless part
of the country. Accordingly, he issued an appeal to those of his
friends who were more happily situated, and eventually his en-
treaties were answered by the totally unheralded arrival of a fine
pair of beavers, escorted by a sceptical Railway Express man.

The beavers had arrived, as beavers will, after all the technicians had gone home; and our colleague was at once placed
in some difficulty, for the animal house was shut and he had no
key. However, he is a man of some resource, and he remembered a disused bathtub up in the attic. He had no first-hand
knowledge of the care and maintenance of beavers in bathtubs,
but he had a vague idea that they would be happier with some
water in the bath, so he dragged it over to a place where he
could fill it from a convenient tap, and brought the beavers up
to admire their new home. Unfortunately the bath had in the
course of time become detached from its plug, and our colleague
cast about for a substitute. Eventually he had a Machiavellian
idea, and retrieved a large carrot from a bag of food outside the
animal house. With this he plugged the bath, partly filled it with

water and tipped the beavers in, having provided them with some food. This done, he went home, tired but happy, having locked the door on his charges.

We need scarcely proceed further. They *did* eat it; there *was* a flood. In fact, the only unexpected feature of the proceedings was that the professor's desk was so nearly vertically under the bath. The resulting interview was full of physiological suggestions, and at its close our friend found that rats would suit his purpose equally well.

Escapee

AN anatomist friend of ours underwent a testing experience the other day. He was sitting in his room doing whatever anatomists do when they disappear from the dissecting-room, when a scrabbling noise made him turn round to observe, sitting on the bench beside his microscope, a large monkey. In the psychiatric and occult literature such an occurrence is, of course, scarcely worthy of comment, but the general run of exteriorised monkeys tend to be small and malignant, with portions of the background furniture showing through. This animal was a ponderous and apparently well-disposed macacque; moreover, it appeared to be pregnant—a circumstance hitherto unrecorded of exteriorisations. Anatomists lead a sheltered life, but they are not devoid of resource: hastily connecting his open door with the repairs to the animal-house along the passage, our friend reached gently for the telephone and informed the animal-man of the whereabouts of his charge.

The cautious arrival of heavily breathing reinforcements, armed to the teeth with nets and poles and sacking, was accomplished outside the door without incident until an injudicious spectator dropped something and swore. At once the placid mother-to-be was converted into a grey blur travelling at great speed round the walls and dislodging copious showers of reprints, boxes of slides, and an anencephalic fetus. The blur eventually shot past our friend's head on to the floor and ran unexpectedly between the feet of the posse to a refuge on top of the large steriliser in the passage. Here it instantly regained its maternal placidity and benign appearance.

By this time there was a large gallery, and much advice was freely given and freely rejected. The embryologist devised an ingenious trap of sacks and netting to be released by a piece of string on the approach of the monkey—a consummation which did not eventuate. A visiting physiologist, armed with a large silk handkerchief, climbed confidently on top of the steriliser, but was swiftly outmanoeuvred and fell, spraining his ankle. The anthropologist, who had been to America, demonstrated the technique of the *bolo* with a string bag to which he had tied two small cabbages, and the neurohistologist used a net and pole and landed some challenging lunges on the spectators. The proceedings were terminated when the animal, mildly irritated, took a leap for a totally inadequate electric light and fell squarely into an open food-bin which our friend (a mere topographist) had the presence of mind to close.

Insect Psychology

A clinical education undoubtedly predisposes to a narrow preoccupation with purely human problems, but glimpses of the larger life keep breaking through. Only the other day our attention was diverted to a letter in *Nature* advocating A Simple Method for Sexing the Confused Flour Beetle. Speaking personally, we had always thought of flour beetles as brisk purposeful creatures, and it is vaguely comforting to learn that they are subject to doubts and hesitancies much as we are, and about much the same subject too.

Now we come to think of it, perhaps this is what is wrong with all insects; this is the tragedy that explains the aimless buzzing on the window pane, the dispirited cockroaches in the scullery. This is what underlies the dry flutterings in the wardrobe, the forlorn cobwebs on the ceiling. They are all confused, poor things, and a good sexing would soon set them right. All except the ants and bees, that is; they have sublimated their difficulties in a thoroughly nasty inhuman way, and we cannot help feeling that they stand in no need of help, or even sympathy.

Bat Hunt 1

IT recently became clear to us that humanity would be benefited
if we could procure a bat to further our researches (a *fledermaus*,
not a willow one), so we set about getting one. We know a
zoologist who lives in the wilds— in one of those places where
a single full-throated 'Ar' is a strenuous evening's conversation—
and arrives at the lab. with burrs sticking to his trousers. He had
lately obtained a green lizard for one of our colleagues; the very
man, we said, to get us a bat.

He proved unexpectedly diffident; he was not, it seemed, that
sort of zoologist. 'How do I catch them?' he said. We explained
that all he had to do was lure the bat into a room and play to
it a record of the ultrasonic squeaks of other bats, thereby
upsetting its echo-sounding apparatus and causing it to collide
with the chandelier and fall senseless to the ground; we had
read it up. He was still not convinced. 'Where do I get the
record?' he asked feebly. 'My dear chap,' we said, 'don't bother
us with details: buy a Galton whistle, ask your air-raid warden,
use a butterfly net, what do we care?'

All this was some time ago, and we still have no bat. We
see the zoologist now and then, but the affair marches badly—
the bats fly too high for him, he says. 'Well,' we replied
impatiently, 'get us a water bat then; they fly only a few feet
up.' He has no water, it seems. We have suggested a tour
of the neighbouring belfries, but he is a Nonconformist
zoologist, on poor terms with the local High Church vicars.
There are no caves in his district either. 'What about barns?'
we said, 'England is an agricultural country, isn't it?' (By this
time we were rather bitter.) But it is no good; his heart is
not in it. 'Too wet for them to fly,' he muttered sullenly when
we passed him in a corridor the other day. We have tried
rehearsing to him a night we once spent in the jungle in the
middle of a rookery of several thousand flying foxes, and
telling him of a Cambridge undergraduate who collected college
bats for dissection. But he isn't shamed. 'You can't expect
them to come out this bright sunny weather,' he told us yesterday.

Does anyone need a green lizard? We know a zoologist who
could get him one.

Bat Hunt 2

THOSE readers who have been troubled by our inability to obtain a bat should take heart; matters are now in train. We did what we should have done at first, and approached our Animal Man. Animal Man, we said (rather diffidently, for we rarely penetrate so far into the animal-house); we are anxious to secure a bat. Yes, sir, he said, laying down his copy of Stephen Potter (he is an advanced Lifeman), what species had you in mind? But we were ready for him. Oh, we said airly, either a Vespertilionid or a Rhinolophid—it's really immaterial. He took it well. Within ten minutes we had learnt both the sporting and unsporting methods of shooting bats, how to bring them to the ground with a long bamboo cane, and the correct technique of trapping them in an old felt hat advanced stealthily over their sleeping bodies. Within half an hour we had ruled out the local church towers because of the swift census. (How's that again? we inquired. Because of the census of swifts, he said pityingly.) Within an hour we had arranged an excursion to a church he knew of where the vicar was Troubled with Bats. Indeed, the ecclesiastical authorities had taken the desperate step of placing in the belfry two stuffed owls to arouse doubts in the minds of the bats. There they still were, said the Animal Man, and uncommonly sheepish they look, if such a term can be applied to stuffed owls.

We set off with light hearts, armed with a rat cage, a sack, a powerful torch, and some leather gloves as a protection against bat-scratch fever. The church was small and whitewashed, and the roof timbers irregular enough to hold a profusion of bats; perched insecurely on the wall were the stuffed owls, putting as nonchalant a face on it as possible. We searched the lower levels systematically, hunting for guano between the pews and the walls, shining our torch inquisitively under the base of the pulpit, and carefully examining the bottom of an empty brandy bottle. We found traces of many pigeons, but no bat spoor; so we retired to the farm to borrow a ladder to inspect the higher reaches of the chancel. Here we struck a snag; the ladder was at present preventing the egress of a number of large and active pigs, and it appeared that the difficulties of our bat-hunt were as nothing to those of the pig-hunt that would result if the animals ceased, even temporarily, to be confined. We learnt that Incense is Best for Bats, but also that we had underestimated the bat-repellent activity of the stuffed owls. It was doubtful if even a single bat remained. Crestfallen, we withdrew to collect our impedimenta, touching our hats respectfully to the owls as we left.

We are still on the trail. Specimens are being reported to us from distances up to 15 miles, and only yesterday we heard of a house in Eire where 300 bats were caught last year. Our travel grant might just run to that.

Plastic Cow

WE are always delighted to chat with our academic colleagues, and the other day when we met a preclinical friend of ours emerging from an unfamiliar building we were at pains to draw him out. It appeared that he had accepted the offer of the department of Agriculture to put him up temporarily while repairs were being carried out in his own department. Our friend is a shy man, and stands somewhat in awe of his adopted Professor, in whom many years of agriculture have matured an already hearty personality. Initially, therefore, our friend viewed his translation with some misgiving, and he was comfortably reassured to observe, standing in the entrance hall of the department, a fine brindled cow of about 2½ hands, entirely composed of some plastic material, and bearing on its face an expression of disinterested benevolence.

For a few days the matter went little further, and beyond nodding to the animal as he passed, our friend made no effort to ripen the acquaintance. One afternoon, however, as he conversed uneasily in the hall with his formidable host, a chance glint of sunlight revealed that the dorsal portion of the cow, including the tail, was detachable. Our friend's knowledge of cows is undeniably sketchy, and it came to him that his horizon would be considerably enlarged could he but remove the detachable portion and investigate what lay within. Clearly, however, the moment was inopportune, and the next day he was at pains to choose a time when nobody was about. The catch was a little stiff, and our friend was injudicious enough to give it a smart tug. With a resounding clatter the cow over-balanced and fell to the floor, retaining its benevolent expression but scattering plastic viscera in all directions. On all sides doors opened inquiringly, and our friend found himself surrounded by a crowd of interested and helpful agricul-turalists.

Nothing was ever *said*, our friend tells us, but the cow has now been moved to the Professor's room, and he feels that the agriculturalists are watching him.

Resident Dog

LAST week we went to cadge a cup of coffee from a geriatrician friend, and were surprised to find, on all the entrances of his empire, the words: *Resident dog in unit: keep automatic doors shut.* We had heard of dogs visiting old people's homes to cheer them up and lower their blood pressure, but had never encountered one that had taken up clinical medicine as a profession. We were eager to learn, and Sister, in her capacity as dog-handler in chief, was happy to enlighten us. The resident dog, she said, had been acquired for a peppercorn rent. It accompanied the staff nurses on their daily drug rounds, and for the remainder of its working hours it was on call either at the nursing station or in the day room. Outside exercise and excretory function were under the control of the nursing staff, but certain trusties among the patients were permitted to perambulate it in the corridors as desired. Though no controlled trials had so far been initiated, the regimen was subjectively considered very successful, apart from the tendency of patients to hand out goodwill titbits abstracted from their rations or their lockers. In America, said Sister rather wistfully, such evil doing is punished by denying the offenders access to the canine therapist.

At our request the resident dog was flushed out from under-neath a table where several patients were enjoying tea and biscuits, and came to elevate our mood and take a few points off our blood pressure in the corridor. It proved to be a low-slung yellow animal of indeterminate ancestry but amiable dispo-sition, and it seemed to take its responsibilities very seriously, especially in the matter of biscuit crumbs. No doubt it hoped to be promoted to the status of registrar dog in the not too distant future.

If canine therapy is here to stay, it may be that a two-tier system will develop, in which insolvent NHS patients will be prescribed generic dogs, while patients able and willing to pay may be allotted borzois, salukis, and the like. Postgraduate diplomas in dog administration will certainly follow, and research projects will seek to determine such matters as the possible therapeutic superiority of soft silky ears over sharp pointed ones. It is but a short step to the provision of distinction awards for dogs, and our own spaniel is thinking of taking the thing up as a career.

The Healing Art

Monkey Therapy

IT is a source of continual humiliation to me that I cannot learn the dosage of penicillin. Only yesterday they came and told me that one of the monkeys was sick and asked me to write out a prescription for it. 'Penicillin,' they said, 'that's what it needs.' If only they had said quinine, now, or morphine, or mag. sulph., I would have had a firm grip on the situation.

The fact is, I am a pre-penicillin man. When I did pharmacology it was at the feet of a muscular and hearty preceptor who insisted that morphine and mag. sulph. were the only two drugs a doctor needed. But even in those happy days my security was being undermined by the manufacture of 'Prontosil' or some such insidious stuff (I never did find out the dose of that either).

I am a dead loss to the drug houses. Every morning a shiny surrealist picture arrives advising me of the passing of yet another pharmaceutical milestone—the *safe* brand of succinylcholinesterase anhydrazine—but I no longer even turn pale. At the mention of phenobarbitone something stirs dimly in my subconscious, but it goes again directly. I can see that my family despise me. When they decide they need a tonic they look at me contemptuously and say 'I suppose it's no good asking *you*, is it?' before they dash along to the chemist. They are quite right, it isn't.

Come to that, I am a pre-electrolyte man too: there wasn't all this nasty sodium about when I was a lad. But then again, when I studied medicine people had their own blood-groups and stuck to them, and you could smoke all you wanted without the statisticians getting at you.

All this, of course, is sour grapes. I envy whole-heartedly those gifted souls who can dash off an illegible 'rep. mist.' with a flick of the wrist in the full confidence that the chemist won't ring them up and have a pained little chat with them.

Chemists always ring me up, even about the monkeys. I can picture them sniggering away to themselves behind their green and red bottles before they dial my number. 'About that prescription, doctor', they say apologetically, 'it's for three times the lethal dose . . . I thought perhaps I'd better check with you . . .'

It is possibly just as well that my therapeutic practice is now confined to monkeys. But I wish they didn't always need penicillin.

Whooping Cough

ONE of our favourite relaxations from the strain of academic life is the study of the weekly statistics of infectious diseases. 'Lot of measles about,' we say, shaking our head knowingly; 'bad year for dysentery too; these poor clinical chaps are having a bad summer.' We click our tongue over the enteric figures, and speak in hushed tones of the decline in scarlet fever. Recently, however, a new emotion has been added; we have a quiet pride in the whooping-cough returns. Remember that sharp spike a couple of weeks back? That was us. Right above the maximum figures for the last ten years we went, just like that. As the spasm shakes us in the night and we rush our asphyxiated stomach to the basin, it is a consolation to know that we have made history.

And not only that—we are learning a lot of clinical medicine too. Both the baker and the man who brings round the lemonade tell us we should go round by the gasworks every day—the smell of the gas always stops the vomiting. The butcher favours blowing into a bottle—it fixed up his partner's niece proper. But the fellow who really impressed us was the milkman. He knows somebody who got a prescription that took the cough away from their kids in no time. 'All you do is ask the chemist for that stuff that tastes like onions,' he told us, 'you'll be right in a jiffy.'

The Right Doctor

ONE day in the pride of my first house-appointment I overhead a stout lady confide to Sister in a hoarse undertone 'Ah want tae see a right doctor. Thon's jist a laddie.' This balanced judgment, I found, merely crystallised into words a fairly general feeling, and many of my associates have subsequently been troubled by the suspicion that I may not, in spite of my now advancing years, be a right doctor. Since I embraced academic life the suspicion has, for most of them, hardened into a certainty. To the layman, the idea that anyone could voluntarily take such a manifestly wrong turning is a strange one. 'Do you mean people call you Doctor?' they ask, over the weekly bridge table. 'Oh,' they say, 'how odd.' And a little silence falls, while they glance furtively at the leather patches on my elbows and then stare speculatively at their own husbands. When they get home they tell each other how sad it all is.

The neighbours have given us up professionally long ago. When we first moved in they used to send their children round, attracted by the prospect of a free medical service just over the fence, and a stand had to be taken. 'You see, he's not that kind of doctor,' my wife explained, 'he does research.' 'Oh,' they said doubtfully, 'really?' It is only too clear that they don't believe a word of it. They have agreed on a harmless convention whereby they refer to me as Doctor when they think I may be listening, and as Mister when they are reasonably sure I am not.

Such a reaction does little to alleviate my own distrust of my rapidly receding clinical acumen. As a student I once cut myself badly during an access of zeal for the study of anatomy, and confidently approached my preceptor, an anatomist of twenty years' standing, loaded with higher degrees and fellowships. 'Oh yes,' he said hesitantly, peering into the spurting depths, 'that's a nasty one; you'd better see a doctor.' With what scorn did I relate this tale to my friends, for from whom should one expect surgical treatment if not from an F.R.C.S.? The other day came retribution. One of the lab. assistants, in the course of an argument with our still, burned his forearm slightly and exhibited the lesion to me. 'Oh yes,' I said hesitantly, 'that's a nasty one; you'd better . . . ' 'No,' I said, 'on second thoughts, reach me down the first-aid box.' He is still alive, and in the limited sphere of the lab. there is a growing feeling that I may, despite appearances, be a right doctor after all. Only yesterday our histological technician asked me if I would pierce her ears.

Non-directive Therapy

A friend of ours had a disturbing experience the other day. She has a small boy who has been in trouble at school, and she went along to seek the advice of a child psychologist to whom she was recommended. Marshalling her facts, she gave the psychologist a masterly outline of the inception and history of the situation, touching on all its ramifications and indicating possible lines of inquiry. The psychologist listened courteously, with his pencil poised between his fingers in a psychological manner. At the conclusion of our friend's account he tilted back his chair judiciously and spoke. 'Well, so you think you have a problem?' he said, and waited. Our friend was a trifle dashed, but gamely repeated her reasons for this belief. 'You certainly seem to be in trouble,' said the psychologist, and began to doodle on the blotting-pad. The silence finally became oppressive, and our friend intimated that she would like some advice. 'Oh,' said the psychologist, 'I don't give *advice*, I'm only here to listen; you work out your own solution. I mustn't interfere with or attempt to guide your own deliberations. It's called non-directive therapy.'

Forced Respiration

THE girls who run our respiratory physiology laboratory are charming in casual converstaion, but when on duty they become stern taskmistresses. Their battery of five formidable machines all possess flashing red lights, and some have electronic readouts of the current stocks of helium, nitrogen, and carbon monoxide in their bowels. The sessions begin with a patient seated at each machine, accompanied by his own personal slavedriver. In every case the patient's duties involve *blowing*, and when the game starts a cacophony of exhortations reminiscent of the labour room rend the air. 'Push! push! push! get it all out! use your tummy muscles, last little bit, go on, push!' The slightest deviation from maximum effort results in a terrifying tongue-lashing, and among the cowed patients foreheads sweat, hernias start from their sockets, and intracranial aneurysms bulge and sway. It is not for nothing that one of the machines is labelled Expirograph.

When the inquisitors are satisfied that their charges have no more air left in them there is a game of musical chairs, each victim and his keeper moving one place to the right. At last there are no more machines to conquer, and the patient is ejected into the corridor in a state of collapse, to be resuscitated by the once again charming technicians with a cup of coffee and a biscuit, such as is provided for blood donors (who do not have to work a quarter as hard). Meanwhile the machines begin a ghastly clicking and groaning as their computers analyse gases, select the best performance of each patient, and print out the results. They find reproducing the graphs particularly distasteful, and express their disgust by a minatory roaring noise.

Eventually the computers fall silent and the five patients are admitted one by one to the Presence, where their mundane symptoms are discussed in the shadow of the unarguable mathematics.

Personally, I feel the best bit is the coffee and biscuit.

The Sluice

THE morning conversations in the spongebag-carrying queue of my fellow patients outside our sluice, though instructive and entertaining, are conducted under certain difficulties. The Noses, who are for the most part completely obstructed by yards of gauze packing, are not always wholly comprehensible, and the Ears, whose audiograms often leave something to be desired, have interpretative problems. As for the Throats, they are sometimes too hoarse to contribute more than a vigorous nodding.

The main topic at such meetings is similar to that common outside the toilets of long-distance aircraft: 'What can they be *doing* in there?' But other matters, such as the progress of the staff-nurse's romance and the propriety or otherwise of sneaking into the sluice after lights out for a quick drag at a cigarette, are disposed of without fear or favour. So is the unreasonable nightly disturbance caused by an elderly farmer, who calls his cattle home, in stentorian tones, at about 3 a.m.

Our doyen is naturally the longest-stay patient, one George, who has been in the ward for an untold number of weeks. We don't like to ask him what has actually been done, but it is rumoured that his sinuses have been taken out and scraped and put back again. In spite of this ordeal he is remarkably spry, and an authority on all matters of hospital protocol and behaviour: he sits at the head of the table at meal times, and helps to dispense the soup. The pecking order among the rest of us depends on the number and nature of the investigations we have undergone. Those who have had a CAT scan are well regarded, but, perhaps strangely, find themselves a step lower than those who are giving off gamma rays following a visit to the department of Nuclear Medicine. (There is nobody in the ward at present who can recount to us a brush with nuclear magnetic resonance.) Those who have been subjected to mere steam radiography, however complicated, rate pretty low, and do well to proffer their opinions cautiously.

I am being discharged tomorrow, and I shall miss our vigorous dissection of local and national affairs. Beginning the day with radio or T.V. will lack the personal touch that togetherness outside the Sluice room brings!

Insomnia

THERE was a time when we used to walk into our chemist's as bold as brass and write ourselves a prescription for sixpennyworth of barbiturate, but since the finger was laid on the barbiturates and benzodiazepines we slink in through the sidedoor after looking round twice to make sure the street is clear. And even once inside our confidence is gone, and we bite our fingernails and look at our watch instead of reaching confidently for the prescription pad. We are not sure any more which hypnotic we ought to take. We made out a time-table recently to see whether we were the type that can't *get* to sleep, and needed rapid action, or whether we *wake* early and should use a longer-lasting affair. Unfortunately we really can't decide, so here it is, and perhaps someone can help us.

2300 hrs. Finish reading improving and soporific Pelican: light out.

2305 hrs. Wife initiates stimulating conversation *re* finance.

2330 hrs. Stimulating conversation ended: wife snoring peace-fully.

2345 hrs. Financial position serious.

2350 hrs. First guest leaves party two houses away: merry laughter.

0010 hrs. Small daughter in tears: rescue expedition. Quote I want you to take my dolly out of my bed and put her on the floor unquote.

0025 hrs. Second guest leaves party: perseverative slamming of car doors: car requires new clutchplates.

0040 hrs. Third and final guest leaves: hosts set out for brisk walk with excited dogs.

0105 hrs. Financial position desperate.

0135 hrs. Starlings in chimney start prolonged fight threatening immediate descent into room.

0215 hrs. Small son coughing hysterically in next room: rescue expedition. Quote my throat tickles unquote. Drink of water.

0235 hrs. Coughing continues: further rescue expedition: after twenty minutes' search find small daughters's cough linctus in boot cupboard: dead wasp on cork.

0256 hrs. Return upstairs: coughing stopped: small son asleep: what about Australian income-tax?

0320 hrs. Six-engined bomber flies over house twenty feet up. Quote what was that noise Daddy unquote.

0321 hrs. Coughing begins again.

0350 hrs. Sudden violent wind (force 7): doors slam, blind vi-brates, photographs swept off dressing-table: break.

0355 hrs. Shut windows.

0425 hrs. Dead calm: suffocatingly hot.

0515 hrs. Birds waken small daughter: carol service on landing.

0525 hrs. Carols waken small son: train noises.

0630 hrs. Children downstairs fighting: begin refreshing sleep.

0705 hrs. Loud knocking: cries of 'Post': registered sample requiring personal signature: wild screams of excite-ment: contents new hypnotic.

A Trying Day

THE latest issue of the *Journal of the Medical Defence Union* includes a list of inquiries received by the M.D.U. during the twelve months which were judged to fall outside the range of matters it should handle on behalf of its members. All of them were redirected elsewhere. The list referred to the following incidents and circumstances:

1. Hitting a policeman.
2. Speeding at 103 mph on a motorway.
3. Drunken driving.
4. Domestic parking dispute with neighbour.
5. Member's own divorce and custody proceedings.
6. Member's theft of 70p from a telephone box.
7. Debt collection of unpaid private fees.
8. Making own complaint regarding a relative's hospital care.
9. Planning application.
10. Income-tax assessment.
11. Domestic burglary.
12. Vandalism of car while parked in school playground.
13. Recommendation of private solicitor for non-medical problems.

As it happens, we know the chap who made the inquiries. They arose in relation to a routine professional visit to a retired schoolmaster, immobilised with arthritis, in a village seven miles along the motorway from the surgery.

Our acquaintance, at times an irascible man, had been put in a bad temper that morning by the arrival of an outrageous income-tax assessment, together with a letter from his lawyer about his impending divorce. He decided to call at the lawyer's office on his way to see the patient, and to take with him his copy of planning proposals for a new lavatory complex for the use of his patients, over which a dispute had arisen. His mood did not improve when he found that his study had been broken into during the night, and that his portable typewriter and his home computer had been taken; the desk had been ransacked, and the plans were nowhere to be seen.

After finishing the afternoon surgery he left on his mission, only to find his car boxed in, not for the first time, by the intrusive parking of his next-door neighbour. After some pretty violent backing and filling, which dented both cars, he drove in a fury to the lawyer's office, where he rapidly formed the opinion that the firm was quite incapable of understanding the iniquity of his wife, who was claiming custody of his only son, and wholly unfit to cope with the criminal negligence of the agency he employed to collect bad debts from his private patients. It would be madness to entrust them with the legal side of the lavatory plans, and as he drove along the motorway he resolved to consult a new firm for all his future problems.

When he arrived at his patient's house it was to find that he had been taken away two days ago to live with his daughter; nobody knew where they had gone. Our acquaintance went to the nearest telephone box to ring his secretary in case she might know the daughter's address, but the phone was out of order. As he left the box he noticed a small pile of money, 70p in all, left on the shelf by a previous frustrated caller. Conscience is the still small voice which warns us that somebody may be watching, and he took a good look round before pocketing the money—as seemed his due in the circumstances.

Outside, he had a better idea, and drove to the village school, where his patient had taught, to ask if they could help. School had finished for the day, but one or two boys were kicking a football round as he parked the car in the playground. The headmaster was delighted to see him, and invited him to take a wee dram in his study. It transpired that the daughter's address was not a quarter of a mile from our acquaintance's surgery, and so overcome was he on hearing this that a further dram became necessary. This led him to ventilate his wrongs to a sympathetic audience, and eventually he recollected yet a further grievance, and discoursed with feeling on the atrocious indignities suffered by his cousin, a patient in the local cottage hospital, where the headmaster served as a member of the board.

By the time he left it was several drinks later, and in the interim one of his tyres had been slashed and one of his headlights kicked in by the young gentlemen who had been playing football. The faint haze which had formed in front of his eyes turned to a sombre red, and somewhat unsteadily and with gritted teeth he changed the wheel.

It was getting dark as he drove back on the motorway, taking his rage out on the accelerator pedal. Unfortunately the police had a speed trap in operation, and he was tracked at 103 mph and stopped. As he now smelled strongly of alcohol, the officiating policeman produced a breathalyser. This was the last straw. Our acquaintance surged from the car and struck the policeman a powerful blow in the stomach.

Next day, out on bail on charges of speeding, drunken driving, resisting arrest, and assaulting the police in the performance of their duties, he spent several hours framing a letter to the Medical Defence Union; it was quite late when he had recovered sufficiently to visit his patient.

Alternative Medicine

SOME time ago I revisited the parish of Little Loch Broom, where I was stationed temporarily during the war. I used to lend a hand with the local sick, and often a box of illicit eggs (the rationing introduced by the English oppressors did not hold in these parts) would be deposited as a fee in the back of the utility by unseen hands. These eggs were never mentioned; such matters were not discussed between gentlemen.

Naturally I got to know the district nurse quite well. At the outset of her ministrations, she told me, she had been the object of a natural distrust, being a foreigner from the next glen, fully thirty miles away. But after some months of enforced inactivity a more than usually daring crofter brought along her first patient, a cow that had broken off one of its horns. She dressed the raw and infected stump with ichthyol and glycerine, and the cow recovered. Another long pause ensued while this result was discussed and assimilated. Eventually a still more daring crofter sent along his wife. She also got better, and this too was regarded as a not unfavourable omen; about a year after her arrival some of the men began to present themselves cautiously for treatment.

One of her patients was a farmer who, many years previously, had set out on his horse one winter night to propose to the local schoolmistress. Suddenly a white hare ran out on to the road in front of him, and this made him very uneasy, for everyone knew that white hares were really witches in disguise. But he rode on bravely, with the hare running in front of him, until it disappeared through the gate of the schoolmistress' house. This was too much; he turned his horse and retreated home to permanent bachelorhood, saved by the sign from marrying a witch.

More recently an old lady who was suspected of being another witch had confirmed the suspicion by cursing a bus because it was full and had no room for her. 'You can go!', she cried, 'But I'll be in Inverness before you!' The bus subsequently went into a ditch, and her reputation was secure.

The local therapeutic regimen for an epileptic child laid down that the father had to go, at a certain phase of the moon, to the grave of a suicide—there were several quite handy—and dig up a skull. He had to take the skull home, fill it with water, and give the child a drink out of it. Latterly an effete modern version of this treatment had gained ground, in which it was not considered absolutely necessary to transport the skull; you simply filled it up on the spot and then decanted the water into a bottle which could be taken home and used equally effectively (I do not know who conducted the controlled clinical trials).

Today the excellent road through the district, the modernised hotel at Dundonnell, and the tourist caravans may lead visitors to scoff. But I warn them not to speak slightingly of the supernatural, for the kelpies that still live in Little Loch Broom are easily offended, and may take a horrible vengeance.

Radiotherapy

MANY years ago we acquired a nice walnut radiogram to play Beethoven to us in the long winter evenings. We were satisfied to observe that it had the usual number of mysterious knobs and flashing lights, and was not too haughty to accept our favourite records. It soon became a member of the family, and was always willing to lend a hand at other jobs, such as supporting the coffee tray when we had guests, or acting as a storage cupboard for comics and half eaten oranges. It was therefore a blow to us when we observed signs of a lesion in the centrencephalic system of our old friend. The onset was acute, and the presenting sign was the extinction of a light which used to illuminate the Home Service: this was rapidly followed by a progressive dysarthria, so that announcers and comics became unintelligible. Finally, in the middle of 'My Word', coma supervened, and our radiogram could neither speak nor play to us any more.

The chap came the next day and took a thorough case history, making notes on a special form. After examining the localizing signs he decided to operate at once, and had soon effected a remarkable and complete remission of the symptoms. When he had finished he presented us with his case-sheet, which we signed, retaining one copy for ourselves. It was terse and to the point. *'Nature of complaint'*, said the form: 'Stopped'. (We were instantly reminded of a certificate we once received from a hospital about our lab assistant: *'Suffering from'*, the certificate read candidly, 'Hospitalization').

'Treatment' went on the form: 'Filament pins of 5V4G resoldered'. There followed an itemized account showing the service call charge, time, and materials; there was a receipt signed by the chap himself, and a place for his *Remarks'*. Finally, there was a short section for our own comments, beginning *'Service Man arrived'*: *'Left'*: *'Was work done to your satisfaction?'* asked the form, and what could we answer thankfully but 'Yes'. The next question cut rather deeper: *'Were any promises made?'* We could remember no promises, so we wrote, rather doubtfully, 'No', and finally signed our name, with the time and the date.

This, it seemed to us, was the ideal form for use by the family doctor in the Welfare State, and we sent a copy to our medical defense society. We liked particularly the bit about satisfaction, and brought it to the notice of our own medical adviser.

Exotica

TO a back-room boy, whose occasional tentative forays into the world of prescribing have hitherto been bounded by the staid columns of *MIMS*, it comes as something of a revelation to read the D.H.S.S. proposed list of drugs and other substances not to be available at N.H.S. expense from April 1, 1985. All human life is there, from the peaceful calm of the cloister ('Balm of Gilead', 'Father Pierre's Monastery Herbs') to the hurlyburly of the business lunch ('Tums' tablets, 'Heart Shape' indigestion tablets) and the anxious problems of the nursery ('Snufflebabe' vapour rub, 'Buttercup' baby cough linctus) and school ('California syrup of figs', 'Strengthening mixture').

Had I been a family doctor, when, I wonder, should I have been tempted to prescribe 'Alpine tea' or 'Aveeno' bar oilated? I should have had some idea of the indications for Male gland double strength supplement tablets, and perhaps also for

'Pro-Plus HeVite' elixir, but I would have been baffled by the list of tablets to formulae ranging in random sequence from A10 to A316 and from B006 to B252. There must be a top-secret code book in the basement of the Elephant and Castle, to which only a selected élite of the profession have a key.

I should have welcomed the opportunity to administer 'Indian brandy solution', or, more simply, wines, but I should, I think, have sheered off morning glory tablets and 'Neoklenz' powder. From the purely personal standpoint I regret the passing of malt extract with cod liver oil *BPC*, having in my youth been rescued from inanition by the same material, and certainly nowadays I could do with some 'Vigour Aids' tablets.

It is dispiriting to think of this great list of preparations, unappreciated and unprescribed, jostling each other on the reject shelves, the 'Day Nurse' capsules comforting the 'Night Nurse' cold remedy and the 'Rock Salmon' cough mixture eyeing the 'SkinGlow' capsules with thinly disguised suspicion. I imagine that out of sympathy many family doctors will rush to prescribe the more exotic items before the opportunity to do so on the N.H.S. is abolished and the great iron doors clang shut.

I am particularly upset by the withdrawal of the 'Junior Cab-drivers Linctus', and I can envisage a lobby of junior cabdrivers proceeding six abreast down Whitehall in bottom gear to hand in a protest against the stigma cast on the only solace which makes junior cabdriving endurable.

The Blisters

1986 will go down in history as the year when I first consoli-dated my position in the ranks of those afflicted by multiple pathology, polypharmacy, and sequential referrals. I had made some progress before, what with my asthma, my oesophageal reflux, my spondylosis, and my pulmonary emboli, but the blisters clinched the position.

When they appeared I was on holiday near the hospital where I once worked, so I went to put the bite on one of the derma-tologists, who in his student days had sat at my feet, but fortunately appeared to bear me no ill-will. At the first session biopsies were taken, lips were pursed, and a wait-and-see regimen was instituted. But when the biopsy results came back I was at once bound, admitted to the underground caverns of immunology, fitfully illuminated by immunofluoresence, and stocked with piles of dimly perceived white cells and alphabetically labelled globulins. The dermatologist assumed—as all clinicians do when talking to me—that I was fully acquainted with the very latest advances in his subject, despite the fact that my house job in dermatology was in the days of triple dye. I was subjected to a disquisition of which I understood very little, though it was apparent that the blisters pointed one way and the proteins and the itching pointed another. Oral steroids, Dapsone, allergic reactions, and dietary factors flickered through the air in my direction, but the one horrifying possibility which I understood, only too clearly, to be on the cards was a gluten-free diet.

Obviously the dermatologist had no idea what he was saying so cheerfully and to whom he was saying it. Born and bred in Scotland, raised from birth on scones, cake, fancy bread, and steam puddings, my whole existence hitherto had been that of a glutenholic. For a fortnight after this gypsy's warning I used to wake up sweating in the middle of the night, envisaging life without gluten, and during the day I doubled my gluten intake in order to give me something to remember in the dark days to come.

The crisis passed, however, and the threat was temporarily averted. It now appears that the pharmaceutical industry can fix me up, though reservations have been expressed about the likely effects of the various medications proposed on my present drug regimen and the combinations and permutations of the possible side-effects. Life was never like this when I was a lad, but I suppose I must move with the times. At least I can eat.

Onychogryphosis

I was never much of a one for Togetherness until the other day, when I heard that medical conferences and pharmaceutical companies' product-launches were being held on luxury cruise ships in the Mediterranean.

That night I had a long and complicated dream. It began aboard a great ship nosing its way out of the Vieux Port of

Marseilles, lights blazing, and the Getting to Know You dance
in progress. I found myself a subsidised delegate to a conference
on Onychogryphosis: a National Emergency. From an obscure
corner I watched the glittering throng in full evening dress
with decorations, chains of office, gardenias, and gold-mounted
identification badges with pharmaceutical logos. On the
Captain's right sat the President of the Royal College of Ony-
chogryphologists, and on his left was the senior representative
of the participating drug company.

In my dream the next morning at sea was rough. After the
Keynote Address slow-release antiemetics were distributed by
white-faced junior reps. Few delegates were able to tackle the
seven-course lunch and the ten-course dinner. The first of the
conference sessions that afternoon, on the molecular biology,
biochemistry, and pharmacodynamics of onychogryphosis, was
poorly attended, but the next day the papers on the pathology
and the treatment of the condition by acupuncture attracted a
sizeable crowd and samples of sun-tan lotion were given out.

The drugs displayed at the alcoholic product-launches which
paralleled these and succeeding sessions were naturally mostly
grypholytics, but there were sets of surgical instruments for
dealing with refractory cases, and hypothermia blankets for
onychogryphosis sufferers unfortunate enough to find themselves caught in a snowstorm in the Cairngorns. The belly
dancer who came aboard at Algiers carried in her navel a
star-burst of newly fabricated tranquillisers, and from her
shapely bosom depended two tassels of the latest H_2-receptor
antagonists, which rotated like catherine wheels under the
sparkling chandeliers.

The enormous meals continued, supplemented by bowls of
soup in the morning and hot chocolate in the afternoon. Instead
of betting on the number of miles covered each day the punters
bet on the quantities of antacids and antispasmodics dispensed
by the cynical ship's doctor.

At the concluding Progress and Review session back in
Marseilles, the Secretary of the College was presented with a
matched set of monoclonal antibodies for his inspired organisation of the conference, which had resulted in only five people
delaying the ship when they were lost in the Acropolis and only
two eluding the search parties in Pompeii. It was felt that an
immense amount of valuable information had been exchanged,

and to universal acclaim it was decided that, though no Recommendations were likely to result, the subject was so important that increased Government funding should be requested for a repetition of the cruise next year.

I was quite sorry to wake up in my own bed on a frosty winter morning.

Homes and Inhabitants

The Scoundrels

IN our manic phase recently we determined to buy a house. After a preliminary study of the form in the local newspaper and some dickering with the agents we finally discovered the only house in England we could afford to buy. Even to our untutored eye it was not in the best of condition, and we timidly approached a local builder to give us an estimate of the necessary repairs before we put in our offer.

The builder, a small active man of a despondent turn of mind, threw himself about the house in a frenzy of estimation. On several occasions he drew sparks from the end of his foot-rule. He peered into the attic and rapped the cistern with his knuckles—'Iniquitous, doctor!'; he stamped on the floorboards—'Neglect, doctor, neglect!' and inspected the fireplaces—'That's a thing I cannot *bear*, doctor!' Outside, the standpipes moved him deeply—'Horrible, doctor!'; and he buzzed gloomily around the drains—'It's illegal, doctor, completely illegal!' He mentally knocked down and rebuilt several walls, lowered the washbasin and raised the sink, and finally squeezed himself through a small bedroom window to inspect the scullery roof. What he saw confirmed his worst suspicions—'Ah, the scoundrels, doctor, the scoundrels!' The garage rendered him speechless, and only after walking away did he find strength to shake his head and mutter 'Oh dear, doctor, oh dear!' He brightened at the unmade driveway—'What you want there, doctor, is a load of gravel, not *our* gravel, you understand, doctor, stuff you can roll', but the garden fence shook him again, and he left enveloped in brisk businesslike gloom.

We are once more making a preliminary study of the form in the local newpaper and have reverted to our depressive phase.

Detached Bungalow

I always move from an area in which house buyers are in the ascendant to one completely controlled by sellers, and the financial problems involved bring on an attack of the twitches.

Having rashly undertaken to buy a flat before trying to sell my present house I am in a state of anxiety as the settlement date draws near and there is still no taker for my Delightful Detached Bungalow, set against a backdrop of forested slopes and within easy reach of the supermarket and other village shops. My deteriorating sleep pattern is not improved by the intermittent presence (I believe the appropriate collective noun ought to be a 'suspicion') of surveyors crawling round above my head and under my feet, sticking their sharp little knives into the woodwork as the fancy takes them, and tapping with infallible instinct the one place where the exterior rendering has come away from the wall.

I suppose I should be grateful when they come, since it indicates that interest in the Detached Bungalow is not yet extinct, but I still find it stressful to answer the surveyors' penetrating questions about damp patches and ceiling cracks, and to watch them writing disparaging comments in their notebooks. One of them found a footrule in the recesses of my foundations and a golfball in the ceiling lagging. Under pressure I was obliged to confess guiltily that I could not explain either circumstance. Another, after telling me with a light laugh that I had a 'dip' in my roof, called for a structural engineer to give a second opinion. This chap arrived yesterday, and eventually passed the roof as fit for seagulls to sit on and the purchasers to shelter under. My outpouring of relief led me to offer him a cup of tea and a piece of shortbread. Mellowed by this lavishness, he asked where I was moving to.

'Oh yes,' he said when I told him. 'We did those flats not long ago. They would be very nice, too, except for . . . ' Here he remembered who he was talking to, and professional reticence stopped him in his tracks. Despite frantic urging, he would say no more. What horrors shall I experience when I move next month—with the Detached Bungalow still unsold?

The Mortgagor

WE were told the other day that one of our colleagues had recently become solely seised in fee simple in possession of a messuage or dwelling-house situate in a piece or parcel of land except and reserved and subject if and so far as mentioned in the First Schedule attached hereto but otherwise free from incumbrances. We are always glad to hear of anybody getting on in life, and we determined to pay him a visit. We found our colleague—hereinafter described as the Mortgagor—precariously established with his family in a bridge-head in the dining-room, the rest of the house being given over to the activities of carpenters, plumbers, carpet-fitters, plasterers and electricians. The Mortgagor's nerves were in poor shape, and as one of the floorboards in the stair succumbed to the electricians with a tearing crash he winced visibly. Between the blows of a sledge-hammer demolishing a party-wall somewhere in the background he confided to us that he had awakened sweating at 2 a.m. for three nights running in the firm apprehension that the dry rot in the kitchen had spread to the bedroom floor and that the bed was in imminent danger of making a sudden descent into the living room. That morning a hamster belonging to the Mortgagor's dependants had escaped from its cage and had eaten a large hole in the new haircord carpet in an attempt to undermine the foundations, and only a few moments ago the Mortgagor had had words with the carpet-fitter, who was now sullenly engaged in sawing a totally unnecessary inch off the bottom of a bedroom door in order to create a draught. Here the Mortgagor's wife produced a cup of tea made with the aid of the painter's blowtorch, and the Mortgagor sipped it moodily. It appeared that there was a peculiar smell in the bedroom, which nobody but the Mortgagor and the Mortgagor's wife could smell, and indeed when we were invited to smell it later we too aligned ourselves with the multitude. There were three dead sparrows in the cold-water tank, and a hornets' nest in the chimney. The curtains belonging to the Morgagor's wife fitted nowhere, and there was a loose board in the dining-room on which the Mortgagor's small daughter was wont to jump up and down, shattering valuable china and completely demoralising the grandfather clock. The Mortgagor stared morosely out of the window at the Timber he had undertaken to preserve; there was a sickly lilac bush close to the house, and we could see it worried him. We inquired with diffidence if there was not perhaps a bright side to the strain of owning a Gentleman's Country Residence, and after some hesitation the Mortgagor admitted that at last he had acquired the style he wanted to write a book on operative surgery. He showed us a specimen page dealing with appendicectomy, which read as follows:

1. Pull and draw opening in lower part of right-hand abdominal wall.
2. Remove and credit appendix.
3. Generally make out with new finishing internally, all to match existing.
4. Reconstruct abdominal wall to detail.
5. Make good surrounds and leave all perfect.

Fred

IN one of our wild moments recently we cast aside our Scottish caution and bought ourselves a new fitted bedroom carpet. Yesterday they sent Fred to lay it. There are few houses in the district to which Fred has not been called at one time or another, for he is seventy, and he has been fitting carpets since he was fourteen. He knows us well. 'Hae ye sellt yer auld pink een?' he shouted as soon as he got inside. 'Yes!' we yelled back into the formidable amplifier Fred keeps strapped round his middle to maintain his liaison with the outside world. He nodded agreement. 'It was sair tashed,' he roared. We did not venture further conversation, for Fred is fond of a pint, and as we intended to stand him one when he had finished; our breath would be needed later. We led him up to inspect our prize. 'Ay, well,' he said consideringly, in tones that shook the plaster, 'she's no a bad carpet!' (Carpets, like ships , are always feminine). We left him to it, and for an hour or so we could hear him bumping around upstairs and clearing his throat with a menacing growl at intervals. Fred works on a sort of echo-sounding principle; whenever he approaches a wall he clears his throat and the resulting concussion tells him how far he still has to go.

When he had finished we took him down the road to the pub, and he told us the news of the day over his pint. It had been a bad one. First he had had a carpet that had been pieced together upside down, so that he had had to go back to the shop and get the lassie to come back with him and take the whole thing to bits and start again. Then he had spent the early part of the afternoon fitting lino in the bathroom of some friends of ours. Fitting lino always renders Fred expansive and he was soon demonstrating on the table with his pint and his pipe. 'Here's the bath here, Doctor, and thonder's the pan,' he thundered, to the interest of the assembled company, 'but I'm no needin' tae tell ye Doctor, ye ken it fine yerself! Twa hoors I wrocht wi' her!' (Bathrooms, like carpets, are always feminine.) To change the subject we screamed an inquiry after his health into the microphone. Fred lowered his voice to a confidential shout. 'It's the screws, Doctor, I get them steady.' Several bystanders nodded understandingly, and murmured sympathetically among themselves. A little knot of people at the far end of the room came closer.

At this point we were unfortunately called to the telephone, and missed the ensuing pathological revelations. When we came back Fred was ready to go home, and the matter had evidently been thoroughly thrashed out. Never mind, we shall get the details when our dining-room carpet comes back from cleaning.

Wasp Hunter

WE met a toxicologist chap the other day, and he told us an exciting story. This chap has never been much of a one for wasps, and when his wife informed him one evening that she had found a wasps' nest in the herbaceous border he was hard put to it to express even a courteous interest. Further conversation, however, elicited the fact that the Little Woman expected him to do something about it. Once the toxicologist chap was thoroughly in the picture he began to draw on his dialectical resources. He was at pains to point out that he had never worked with insects, that his grandmother suffered from angioneurotic oedema, that wasps did little harm, and that it was fatal to approach a matter of this sort in too great haste. 'Well,' said his wife, turning over a page 'something has got to be done, and *I'm* not going to do it.' This ultimatum caused the toxicologist to venture outside to inspect the problem. There was a large hole in the ground, and a constant coming and going of large healthy wasps, each containing several milligrammes of assorted acids and toxins. Several flew round the toxicologist's head, intimating in a sinister buzz just what they would to to him should he come any closer. He retired hastily to complain to his wife that he hadn't any suitable clothing. 'There's an old muslin curtain in the drawer' said his wife curtly, selecting another chocolate; by this time she had her feet up on the toxicologist's chair. A beaten man, the toxicologist apprehensively proceeded to whip together a lethal brew of D.D.T., paraffin, and petrol. He was handicapped by his ignorance of the mean body-weight of the population of wasps, but eventually his mind reverted to the bad old days when he too used to write 'q.s.' on prescriptions and he made up a vast empirical blunderbuss dose. Swathed in anti-wasp clothing, including his demob. hat and the muslin curtain, he boldly poured his mixture down the hole, sealing it with a large stone. There was a dead silence, except for one late-comer plaintively anxious to join its cousins in the holocaust inside, and the toxicologist returned jauntily to the house, well pleased.

Next morning he went to view the battlefield. There was a large stone on the ground, and a constant coming and going of large healthy wasps buzzing reproachfully.

Thus began a toxicological saga lasting five days. Boiling water, cyanide, caustic soda, detergents, coffee grounds, and plant hormones merely increased the ill-will of the wasps without affecting their viability. The toxicologist chap laid out all his stock of anti-histamine samples on the front doorstep, just in case, but no-one was stung. Finally he thought of fire, the great cleanser. He poured paraffin down the hole, introduced a burning rag, and retired, as they say on the fireworks. The flames were most gratifying. After a couple of hours or so the toxicologist got tired of watching them and went to bed: at intervals during the night he could see a companionable flicker on his ceiling. By lunch-time the next day their vigour had somewhat abated and he was able to cap the gusher with another large stone. There were several dead moths lying around, but there was not a wasp in sight. Flushed with victory, the toxicologist repaired to his car and was immediately severely stung by a bee which had been taking its siesta on the driving seat.

Worried Gardener

I used to think highly of Spring, but nowadays I am glad when it is over, for it has become a very worrying season.

My parents were enthusiastic gardeners, and when visitors came I was expected to attend ward rounds in the garden and greenhouse. Seedlings would be assessed as small for dates, mineral and hormonal deficiences in the herbaceous border would be diagnosed, and alternative treatments for metabolic and infectious diseases discussed at tedious length. These experiences, like many of those in my clinical course, used to induce in me a hypothalamic cut-off, a *belle indifférence*, which detached me from the real world and led to a lasting antipathy to horticulture. I was a dutiful child, and dug where I was told to dig, mowed when so directed, and watered when higher authority deemed it necessary, but my spirit was elsewhere. As for weeding, I could usually recognise grass, and on my good days nettles, bracken and dandelions as well, but the finer distinctions between noxious invaders and priceless assets remained permanently beyond me.

Now, however, as the unwilling proprietor of a small garden, I am forced by the pressure of public opinion to keep it purged of agents which might contaminate adjacent properties, all maintained with loving care.

I have read enough science fiction to know that there are plants around which, if not immediately exterminated, could spell the End of Civilisation as We Know It, so when the first crops of tiny indeterminate green affairs appear in the borders I overreact and set about them savagely, to be on the safe side. It is only later, when my native hue of resolution becomes sicklied over with the pale cast of thought, that I start waking up at four in the morning. What if these little round leaves belonged to a rare mutant, which would have astonished Chelsea? Or perhaps to a Siberian exotic, brought here on the feet of an avian visitor unknown to science? Or even to a beautiful carpet of protective ground cover, installed at enormous expense by the previous owner? Where is the parsley I planted last year?

One of my neighbours, who speaks with forked tongue, continually compares the barren spaces where nothing grows but cigarette packets and paper bags brought by the wind from his rubbish bin ('everything looks so *tidy*') with the wild riot of overblown colour customary in the days of my predecessor.

This year my nerve cracked, and I gave the garden its head. The willow herb and bracken are thriving, brambles flourish everywhere, and the lupins have suffered a malignant transformation, with secondaries all over the place. Yesterday I swear I saw a thing like a giant groundsel *moving*. But at least I get some sleep, and it is a long time till next Spring.

Caterpillar

IT is only a few days since our caterpillar moved in, but already he dominates the household. He lives in a glass plum-pudding jar beside the goldfish, on the ledge behind the kitchen sink. He will, we are given to understand, eventually become an elephant hawk moth, but that is in the distant future. For the present he is three inches long and proportionately stout, immensely inquisitive but easily frightened. Every time we breathe on him he rolls over and goes into a convulsion. He has, nevertheless, an enormous appetite, and it is this that has been worrying us. He was found on a clarkia, and so far we have managed to sustain him on leaves from the solitary specimen in our garden, which is now almost razed to the ground. We have tried to tempt him with michaelmas daisy, but he thought nothing of that. Lilac leaves gave him a mild gastro-enteritis, and he would not touch chrysanthemum. In the hope that he might have exotic tastes we tried him with nasturtium and mint, but the fumes were nearly too much for his delicate constitution, and we had to take out the leaves quickly. In desperation we looked up a handbook. 'Food-plants,' said the handbook concisely, 'Willow-herb (*Epilobium hirsutum*), Water bedstraw

(*Galium palustre*). Also reported on Enchanter's Nightshade (*Circaea lutetiana*) and various kinds of bedstraws. In captivity,' ended the handbook a trifle censoriously, 'it devours fuchsia greedily.'

So there we are. There is no willow-herb for miles, bedstraw to us is just something we shove into our palliasse, and we don't think that blue thing in the middle of the herbaceous border can be enchanter's nightshade. There remains our fuchsia—a tender and backward plant destined in ten years to be the glory of our southern exposure. We just couldn't do it, not even for a friend. Yesterday, after an impassioned argument lasting well over an hour, we agreed to give him just two leaves, Daddy, only two, to test the veracity of the handbook. When we looked in this morning with our breath suitably bated we found ourselves sharply aligned against the handbook. He had not attempted to eat any fuchsia, and the poor remnants of our clarkia had been insufficient to satisfy him. His head waved at us pathetically. There was only one thing to do. Tonight, after his proprietor was safely in bed, we took him and set his feet stealthily but firmly on the clarkia at the bottom of a garden we know just along the road.

Nocturnal Gardening

As I grow older, my attention span grows shorter, and my wife has a standard solution for my difficulties. 'Why don't you go out and water the lawn?' she says, 'I'm sure you can think better out there than in here watching the T.V.'. Here in Western Australia lawns are valued and water is scarce; in the black times of water shortage lawns sometimes have to be watered by hand between the hours of eight and ten at night, and the opportunity this affords for uninterrupted and consecutive thought could hardly be improved upon. Out there in the scented darkness, lit through the swaying trees only by the yellow street lamps and the splendid Southern moon, what greatness could the mind not achieve? In theory, that is.

Up to date I have composed no sonnets out on the lawn, written no symphonies, formulated no philosophy. When the spray has blown back on me on a gusty night, saturating my trousers, it may be that I have invented a few striking phrases, but my thoughts remain incurably earthbound and my attention incurably disposed to wander.

In our garden the wind drives all manner of things up against our rose bushes, and other, more solid material seems to sprout from the defenceless poppies. One night, for instance, my beachcombing activities produced, in addition to the usual irresistible scraps of letters from unknowns to unknowns, a large placard reading 'Only 60c a dozen', a sticky label with the words 'Sold Dryburgh', and a tag reading, Oxygen 120 cu ft. Specially prepared for medical use'. To a mind as commonplace as mine this sort of thing is fatal. What can you get for 60c a dozen? What did they sell to Dryburgh which so disgusted him that he unstuck the label in the middle of our street? Or was it Dryburgh who did the selling? Who among our neighbours is using oxygen, and what is the matter with them?

There are other diversions. It was from this lawn that I saw the first Russian sputnik the night after it was launched; that was a night for excitement, and the watering was at once forgotten. (Now, they rumble in their dozens above my head, unseen and unattended, familiar denizens of Space). The planes, flashing white and green and red, circling out over the distant sea before coming in to land ten miles away, always distract me from my myriad potential discoveries, for I speculate in what frame of mind those on board are fastening their seat belts and putting out their cigarettes. Excitement at a new country and a new life? Boredom with a too familiar trip? Apprehension? Regret? My heart goes out to the airsick ones who, like myself, are simply thankful to be approaching solid ground.

But even when there is no distraction except the occasional passing of a car and the faint barking of suspicious dogs my mind drifts off on its own. Rather than face the problems of the present and future it wallows gratefully in the past, substituting for the sweetness of gardenia and frangipanni the remembered pungency of broom and heather, for the hiss and splatter of the spray from the wet nozzle in my hand the dripping of rain on beech leaves after a summer shower.

Nostalgia is the curse of Scotland.

The Emigrant

A friend of ours who is thinking of emigrating to Australia has obtained a copy of the property section of a newspaper in order to study the sort of housing available. To someone accustomed to the suave verbosity of British houseagents the advertisements appear somewhat stark. Though many of the adjectives ('superior', 'delightful', 'superb', 'immac.') have a familiar ring, there are none of the tranquillizing flourishes ('The spacious and well-planned accommodation comprises . . . ; magnificently situated in rolling parkland; a real family home for the discerning') on which the profligate British expend their clients' money.

The paragraphs of abbreviations and acronyms in the paper closely resemble the private codes in which the case notes of hospital patients are nowadays written and our friend found it necessary to call in his Australian senior registrar to act as interpreter. It appears that 'bt. 2br.s/o' signifies a brick dwelling with a tiled roof, two bedrooms and one sleep-out (an additional bedroom stuck on the exterior and entered either from the garden or from one of the inside rooms). 'Fc + wt' conveys that the floor coverings and window treatments are for sale with the house, 'BIR' means a built-in (ward)robe, and 'feats' (transl. 'features') is an umbrella term which could shelter such diverse phenomena as a split-level bathroom, a built-in play-pen, or a bar in the master bedroom. 'River view' speaks for itself, and in the process adds some thousands of dollars to the purchase price, while 'river glimpse' indicates that if the proud owner were to climb up on the chimney stack a glint of silver would be visible in the middle distance; this is slightly less expensive.

Outside in the garden, 'bbq' is easy, and 'retic' not very diffi-cult, but 'amens' may, it seems, carry several interpretations of the word 'amenities', from a jacaranda in a neighbour's garden to a drive-in alcohol outlet on the corner. On the other hand 'bgp' is very precise, meaning a below ground (swimming) pool.

Everything sounds so romantic that we are thinking of joining our friend in a triplex with casual lrs., semiensuite WIRs and dbl/1/up garages.

House Warming

WHEN I read the Sunday papers I am at pains to avoid the advertisements for fireplaces and central heating, for the proud smiles on the faces of their ostensible owners irritate me. In my experience heating a house is no smiling matter, and at no time did I ever smirk in this fashion, for I always feared the worst, and was seldom disappointed.

The first coal fire I had under my undisputed control was in a flat in the upper reaches of a tall four-storeyed house built in the days when the mistress could ring the bell in the confident expectation that the Staff would climb the stairs to clear away the tea things and bring up a scuttle of coal. The bell was still there, but the staff was not, for this was just after the war; it was I who had to carry the scuttle up the four flights of stairs from the cellar.

In the appalling winter of 1946/7 I lit the first fire of my married life in this grate, with high hopes of holding frostbite at bay. The paper and the sticks burned briskly, but the dirty grey material on top remained completely inert. For an hour or so I laboured over it before I accepted the fact that to make a fire the fuel must be combustible. I spent the next evening in the cellar sieving the mound of dust representing our ration for the next three months in the belief that I might find something which could catch alight, but nothing I found could be induced to burn. We were driven back on an electric fire which, in the intervals of electricity cuts, charred the fronts of our legs into a pattern of purple blotches, leaving quite untouched the sub-zero atmosphere behind us.

Later on we graduated to a small concrete semi-detached box where the snag was the chimney, for the house had belonged to an eccentric builder with unorthodox views on the construction of chimneys. The flues were so peculiar that only one chimney sweep would tackle them, and he had retired. As a consequence the soot accumulated steadily until the chimney caught fire and cleaned it out for a time; the process then began all over again.

There was a metal inspection plate in the wall of the living room which could be opened with a special key, disclosing the black labyrinth beyond. One afternoon I was sitting in an armchair in front of a bright fire when an enormous roaring noise began and the inspection plate shot across the room, narrowly missing my head and releasing a great vomit of soot on to the carpet. Flames licked out into the room. The neighbours, aroused by the clang, shouted what was obviously practised advice to us through the window. 'Don't get the fire brigade!' they cried; 'the house'll be ruined, and you'll be fined as well'. Meanwhile I had scooped the soot up into a bucket, and was attempting to block the hole with the plate, which proved to be red hot. My wife's hand was on the telephone leading to material and financial ruin when at last the outburst subsided, and eventually all was quiet except for the smell of burning carpet and the black scorch marks on the ceiling.

Our first brush with a modern fireplace occurred in another house, where we decided to install one of these grates with an adjustable draught control, so that at a touch of the knob its contents would spring from gentle hibernation to a roaring life. And indeed this was what actually happened; we were delighted to possess a heating machine which actually worked. But it was curious that when we had the fire on we noticed a considerable wind blowing across the floor from under the door to freeze our defenceless backs. Naturally this was mere coincidence; the fire took its draught from under the floor, for the booklet had told us so. We fitted a draught excluder under the door and sat back confidently. But the keyhole now started to moan in a ghostly fashion, and wind began to leak in round the windows and at the sides of the door. We fitted metal strips to the door, but these proved an irresistible attraction to the local earwigs and the wind through the windows increased to gale force; the fire began to smoke. We cut a hole in the outside wall under floor level to give the fire all the oxygen it needed, and began to have draughts in front of us as well as behind.

After a while we gave it up and decided that we were being fussy and un-British; it was *healthy* to have the different parts of your body at different temperatures. Look at the way all the central heating gave the Americans sinusitis and chills – to say nothing of their appetite for ice-cream, which all the papers told us led to arteriosclerosis. After all, was it not being roasted on one side and frozen on the other that inured our fathers to the rigours of founding the British Empire?

We had some reason to be sceptical of central heating. At one time we had shared a house in the country with four other families; it had an ancient central heating system depending on a boiler which crouched, black and malignant, at the bottom of an almost vertical staircase leading darkly to the cellar. The boiler was always surrounded by a choking miasma of sulphur dioxide, and on the days when it was my turn to clean and feed the monstrosity I used to emerge purple in the face and wheezing. Yet all these superhuman efforts could achieve no more than an erratic trickle of lukewarm water which gurgled through a few of the less accessible radiators scattered through the house. Our wives sat with rugs round their feet, pained, blue, and reproachful.

After yet another move we had under our sole ownership a quite different sort of boiler – split new, with a cream finish which dared us to sully it with anything but the cleanest coke. It sat in the kitchen, and had a regulable air intake which could be adjusted with a screwdriver in the most scientific manner imaginable.

It was about a week later that I carelessly left the door of the machine open a crack one night instead of making sure it had clipped shut. At one in the morning we awoke convinced that the place was on fire. The bedroom was like a turkish bath, and when we staggered downstairs we found the kitchen shaking and heaving in sympathy with the efforts of the boiler, which was glowing red and shuddering. Plaster was falling from the walls through which the hammering pipes left the kitchen. I managed to get close enough to slam the boiler door with the poker, and turned on the taps to let out the steam. All I produced was an unnerving silence; nothing whatever, neither vapour nor fluid, came out of any of the taps for the rest of the night. Next morning, however, the frightened water had returned; where it had taken refuge, I have no idea. It was days before the house cooled down, but the water stayed cold for a week.

When we moved to Western Australia we did not expect, in a state celebrated for its climate, ever to be cold again, and we set about house hunting in the heat of February without much thought of inspecting in detail the heating apparatus which went with the houses on offer. When we finally bought an old house (i.e. built over ten years previously) we paid little attention to our old enemy, the open fire-place. Indeed when we made our tour of inspection, this particular specimen was occupied by a collection of exotic indoor greenery, and we gained the impression that no fire had ever been necessary.

It was not until July that we even thought of a fire. But one morning we woke up feeling rather chilly, and that evening we thought it would be nice to remove the greenery and have a little fire of jarrah logs, just as an experiment. The smoke billowed straight out into the middle of the room − brown asphyxiating stuff, which settled like a scum on every exposed object, staining the walls and ceiling. In spite of all efforts at prevention, it continued to billow for eight years, for electric fires did not touch the swirling masses of cold air which in winter eddied through our open-plan warm house. The chimney ran vertically up towards heaven, unhampered by flues or bends or complications of any kind, and nothing I could do would induce the smoke to prefer this pathway of escape to the alternative one leading across our faces to the windows and doors; I had to paint the ceiling and the fireplace every year, and would have been glad to refit the entire family with a new set of respiratory tubes, if only this had been possible.

Since returning to Scotland we have experienced the most curious device of all − electrical ceiling heating. Under this mad dispensation, flying in the face of schoolboy physics, the temperature near the roof of the living room was a measured 4−5°C more than that near the floor. Cerebrospinal fluid boiled off gently while feet froze in spite of bedsocks and rugs. We were forced to fall back on our ancient free-standing electric fires, which on more than one occasion set fire to our cocker spaniel, and which nowadays cannot be renewed.

I should like to be able to smile like these chaps in the Sunday papers, but the best I can do is to bare my teeth.

Gourmet Manqué

As a teacher of a little-regarded subject in the medical curriculum I have spent most of my life eating institutional food; even the sandwiches at Faculty meetings have always contained ham or mousetrap cheese rather than anything more venturesome.

So now that I have to fend for myself I find that my potential as a gourmet has been irretrievably impaired. In the brief interval before Alzheimer consigns me in a plain van to yet another institution, I simply cannot be bothered to launch out on a gastronomic voyage of discovery.

Nevertheless, as I stand in line moodily clutching my ticket and waiting for the girl to call out 'Number 47: black pudding and chips', I sometimes wonder just what the recipes I read in the glossy magazines would taste like. I mean the sort which begin 'Marinate seven Albanian truffles (all others are too loose in texture) for 22½ hours in a mixture of one part avocado juice to three parts guava vinegar . . . '

The cookery programmes on television result in products easier to imagine, but their main courses tend to involve three-quarters of a bottle of burgundy, and the sweets depend on six egg yolks and a pint and a half of double cream. My wayward stomach, which spends much of its time in my chest, has long ago intimated its opposition to such delicacies, and, furthermore, I reason that all these little gallipots and Petri dishes plated out with unheard-of spices and rare herbs would have to be washed up afterwards.

Accordingly, as I heat up my mince, I tell myself, not for the first time, that mince makes for a longer life than pâté de foie gras or caviar. Whether this is true or not remains to be seen, but at least I can truthfully say that I have been conditioned to enjoy it just as much.

Chop Picnic

DESPITE a lack of corroborative evidence, summer must have arrived, because the chap up the road has set up his barbecue in the back garden. The sight of this fearsome apparatus always reminds me of my introduction, many years ago, to the more basic ritual of the Australian chop picnic.

The principle is simple: you take an ample supply of raw red meat, drive to a spot where the bull ants and the tiger snakes are not too thick on the ground, build a fireplace with the neighbourhood stones, and collect a pile of dry gum leaves and sticks. If you are a dedicated Aussie, you then light the fire by rubbing two sticks together, if not, you use a match. The meat is placed over the flames on a rickety platform made of folded chicken wire and converted into gritty carbon, which you hold in your hand and tear to pieces with your teeth, manifesting every sign of enjoyment. Meanwhile a billy with a wire handle, usually an old tin that once held kerosene or weedkiller, has been filled with stagnant water from the creek and is now boiling. A handful or two of tea is thrown into it at a precise moment determined by divination, a green gum leaf is added to the potion as propitiatory magic, and the whole is then whirled around to distribute the various solids, which by this time include a few bush flies, ants, and perhaps a small lizard. The resulting stiff brown suspension is then drunk, again with every expression of delight.

At first, I was in no position to protest. But after I got married and my wife, who was a strong supporter of this ceremonial meal, began to inflict it on me, I suggested that I might be provided with a small bacon-and-egg pie to eat while I had the pleasure of watching other people appreciate their charred chops. I also put in a plea for a beer or lemonade in place of the curious bitter brown syrup, and I was, rather pityingly, indulged in these whims.

But at least the Australian routine has one great advantage over the effete British one, where paper plates and even knives and forks may be provided. The ambient air is usually warm or hot, whereas attendance at this chap's barbecue up the road means putting on three or four sweaters and taking along oilskins and an umbrella.

Metropolitan Lunch

ONE of our colleagues on rare occasions travels to London to attend meetings, when he usually has a blameless and uneventful midday meal at B.M.A. House. Last week, however, he took his wife with him, and, one thing leading insensibly to another, he found himself having lunch in one of these Temples of Fashion which infest the broader streets of the Metropolis. He was half way through his chicken-and-ham patties (our colleague is not a clinician, and cannot afford to aim high), when he observed that his wife's eyes had narrowed, and turning lethargically round, his gaze encountered that of an exotic raven-haired beauty, liberally besparkled and in full off-the-shoulder evening dress. The beauty executed a couple of brisk pirouettes, and, taking the flounce of her skirt in one hand, swished it smartly at our colleague. After which she smiled radiantly and withdrew, leaving a large central scotoma in our colleague's visual fields. Nothing in his previous experiences at B.M.A. House had prepared him for such a phenomenon, and he spent the rest of the meal in an uneasy state. At intervals he fancied he heard a rustle of taffeta behind him and whipped round at great danger to life and limb only to find the waitress regarding him stolidly. During his steamed fruit pudding he several times felt the hot breath of further exotic beauties on the back of his neck, but investigation disclosed no basis for this sensation, and he left the restaurant without any additional manifestations being vouchsafed.

Nevertheless, the experience has left its mark upon him, and even while sitting in our own canteen he has a tendency to twitch violently and scrutinise the space immediately behind him. He expresses himself as dissatisfied with rural life.

Menu for Halley

THE silly season is usually defined, on a dull political basis, as the months of August and September, when Parliament is in recess. But for me it is bounded by the now traditional twin races to be the first to eat grouse on the morning of August 12 and the first to drink a bottle of the current year's Beaujolais fetched across the Channel in mid-November. In between these dates quantities of what purports to be champagne are wildly sprayed at sporting events, golf balls are hurled into crowds, and cups and trophies are soundly kissed for the benefit of the media.

These customs clearly give innocent pleasure to many people, but most of them leave me cold. I have eaten my share of mildly unusual meat courses, from goat to wallaby via reindeer, water buffalo, and capercailzie. But there is no way I would eat, at an inordinately expensive breakfast, a grouse that had not been

hung before cooking. Nor am I keen to be sprayed with champagne, or hit on the head by a golf ball.

The Beaujolais, though, is a different matter. I have sampled
the wartime mixture of lower alcohols known as North Queensland plonk, and also the material said to have been called Post
Office Red because it was formerly sold in New Zealand post
offices. These trials have rendered me well prepared to sink my
teeth into a bottle of raw Beaujolais, should one be waved in
front of my nose.

In fact, the current extension of the silly season to cover the
visit of Halley's comet gave me the opportunity of designing a
menu for a comet-watching session. Some time ago a young
kamikaze grouse immolated itself against the radiator of my
car, and was consigned to my freezer. Later my dog caught
and proudly presented me with a squirrel. What could have
been a more appropriate accompaniment to astronomical observation than a ragôut of grouse and squirrel, washed down by
Beaujolais nouveau? Even Halley's comet (otherwise in my
book something of a non-event) might thereby have acquired
a rosy glow which would have lingered in the memory. But
alas, the comet spent its time in my region of the Northern
hemisphere shrouded in impenetrable clouds, and unless I take
my celebratory meal with me to Mauritius or the Seychelles,
I shall have to look for another occasion worthy of it.

Cold Comfort

IN one of our wild moments a few months ago we bought a
refrigerator. Not one of these massive jobs we have seen in the
houses of our clinical colleagues, with automatic defrosting
at 3.20 a.m. and a special compartment for caviar; just a small
affair to keep our milk cool. For some time after it came we used
to open and close the door happily, watching the light come on,
but after a while we came to accept cold milk as one of the facts
of life, and even acquired a taste for hard butter. Judge, then,
of our dismay when the other day the refrigerator packed up
and refused to work for us any more. Our sunny disposition
became quite clouded, and we spoke snappily to our youngest
child. Clearly something had to be done, and our scientific

training led us at once to the solution; we rang up the refrigerator chap.

He was not surprised to hear from us. 'I've been expecting this to happen,' he said in a manner reminiscent of surgical outpatients. 'Listen,' said the chap, 'there's only one thing to do. Switch her off and let her cool. Turn her upside down and you'll hear her gurgle. Let her sit for about half-an-hour and then turn her back again. There's a 75–90% chance you'll get good function again; but if not,' said the refrigerator chap briskly, 'you can't expect any function at all.'

We are not very quick on the telephone, and clinical instructions always did confuse us, but eventually the position got across, and we ventured to ask what happened if we got no function. 'Ah,' said the chap with some unction, 'new unit; nineteen pounds, six and eleven.'

We turned her upside down with considerable trepidation, which rapidly changed to black despair when we found she did not gurgle at all. She sat for half an hour in an atmosphere of mounting tension, and when we went back to turn her again we observed to our horror a sullen stream of yellowish sticky fluid emanating from her mechanism. Greatly daring, we inserted an exploratory finger and traced this to its source—a sodden handkerchief containing a quantity of boiled sweets deposited there for safety by our youngest child. We called for our toothed dissecting forceps and disimpacted the offending mass. Immediately our ears were gladdened by a reverberating gurgle of a singularly musical quality. She gurgled contentedly for nearly five minutes and then relaxed into a placid stupor. Confidently we turned her over; we switched her on and off she went. She has given us good function ever since, and we are thinking of inviting our clinical colleagues to an ice-cream conversazione.

Food Parcel

ONE of the chief features of our annual pilgrimage to the North is our visits to the shops. The sweet-shops, for example. In Scotland the buying of sweets is properly recognised for what it is—a serious and important business. As the bell rings the presiding genius emerges from the ben room to discuss our respective healths, canvass our opinions on the weather, and in general initiate a friendly chat on the topics of the day. After some time we gently steer the conversation round to the merchandise on the shelves, and a delightful conducted tour among this ensues, with brief judgments and summaries, assisted in borderline cases by a judicious sample. 'This is mebbe rather a darker chocolate than ye might like': 'These ones have a kind of chewy centre': 'This one is new and I canna just recommend it personally, but it's been selling very well.' Eventually the appropriate mixture of caramels is specially blended for us from several assortments, and we collect our little parcels and leave with mutual assurances of good will.

The same attitude permeates other branches of trade. On our last visit we decided to bring back with us some of the excellent beef we had been eating, and we visited the butcher to arrange matters. We felt at once that we were in good hands. Our problem was gravely and sympathetically received, and it was felt that our needs would best be served by a nice joint from a black bullock which was to be killed the next day. The butcher sketched the pedigree of the bullock for several generations—he was of good Scottish stock. His life had been cut short before his prime, and indeed he had never been away from his mother. In short he was just the bullock to revictual an English household. As we drove south we thought occasionally of the black bullock's sorrowing mother, while the nourishing parcel in its special wrapping swung behind us in the boot. Next morning we opened it up, our mouths watering, and our expectations were not disappointed.

The day after the obsequies were finally completed we went out to buy some English stewing steak. 'No steak,' said the butcher, his gaze fixed on the roof just above our heads. 'Well then,' we said, 'what about some mince?' 'No mince till tomorrow' he said, switching his tongue from one cheek to the other dispassionately. 'Oh', we said, 'good morning', 'Morning,' said the butcher, turning his eyes to the roof above our successors in the queue.

We had come home.

Plastic Trouble

IN appearance and habits we are in no way remarkable, and it has been our ambition to proceed inoffensively through life, breathing quietly through our nose and causing as little fuss as possible. But recent events have conspired to present us to the world as a wrecker, a vandal, a despoiler of other men's property. We are having Plastic Trouble.

The first manifestation of our Trouble occurred while we were on holiday in Devon. We were sitting comfortably one morning on the black plastic seat, placidly admiring the black bath and the lurid murals of orange flames, when we were startled to hear a sharp crack and to have our equilibrium momentarily disturbed. When we looked, what should we find but a comminuted fracture of the left posterior quadrant of the seat. They were very pleasant about it, but we said no, it was entirely our fault, and we must insist on paying (thirty-five bob it cost us, too).

The second manifestation was a couple of months ago, while we were visiting a friend of ours in the pathology department. A nice white job it was, but white or black is all the same to our Trouble, so long as it is plastic, and crack it went just like the first. On this occasion we were slightly less inclined to take an altruistic stand on the matter of payment, but fortunately our friend made little of the occurrence, and we wrote it off to departmental maintenance.

The third attack took place last week, in the newly opened establishment in connection with our hospital library. This time we did not hesitate. As soon as we heard the now familiar crack we made haste to sneak out as unobtrusively as possible, leaving our senior assistant surgeon, the only other occupant of the library, to take the blame.

We find all this very disturbing, and the thought that at any time we must expect to hear the short sharp report marking the end of number four is interfering with our sleep. We had no difficulties of this kind in our youth. We remember a large wooden throne on which we were wont to spend many happy hours singing to the illustrated papers which were stored in lockers on each side of the business portion of the machine. At school the seats were made of inch-thick timber, and in later years we had occasion to patronise a cold stone contraption in a Scottish castle. A man could relax, without fear of personal injury or financial embarrassment, when seats were solid affairs made of natural material and not flimsy wafer-like contrivances whipped up out of coal and air and casein.

The Shower

LAST month, after the four well-spaced telephone calls which are necessary to secure the services of the local plumber, our new and most carefully chosen bathroom shower was installed.

The previous shower, which we inherited with the house, was forbiddingly complex, with levers, dials, and knobs suggestive of the control room of a nuclear power plant; visitors required an intensive series of tutorials before being let loose on it. In our search for a replacement we therefore rejected as too complicated a jacuzzi-like model with multiple taps, and turned our attention to simpler mechanisms. Our experience with other people's showers had included some in which turning the control 2 mm to the right or left altered the ambient microclimate from freezing to scalding, some which could do no more than dribble prostatically, and others which flayed the skin off the shoulders with a high-pressure torrent. We had been subjected to self-extinguishing showers which dried up completely when someone turned on the tap in the kitchen, and to irregularly variable showers requiring constant readjustment during use. We had bitter memories of a shower in which the normal colour coding of the taps was reversed, and of another which developed airlocks in the hot water supply, making it essential to dismantle and invert the system every time before using it.

Bearing all these horrors (and more) firmly in mind we eventually settled, rather doubtfully, for a shower which the leaflet assured us was simple, reliable, and user-friendly (what used to be called 'student-proof'). Indeed, it has proved to be free of the defects we had feared, but destiny is not so easily evaded. When in full-blooded use, our new shower creates an intolerable banging and whistling throughout the house. Dogs howl, the neighbours think the Martians have landed, and the bathroom window has developed a greenstick fracture. In despair we have put through the first two of the statutory four calls to the plumber, and have been reduced to using the bath. This, though less traumatic from an auditory point of view, is, like most modern baths, unsuited to our needs, having been constructed with no thought of accommodating anyone over four feet in length.

Amateur Trichologist

SOME years ago, when we were working with rabbits, we injudiciously bought a pair of electric clippers to facilitate cutting their hair. This apparently put us on the mailing-list of all the hairdressers' suppliers in Britain, and we have been bombarded and even pursued abroad by letters containing special Easter offers to trade in our worn-out scissors or telling us how to get another 3d. or 6d. on every haircut without having to spend any money on extra equipment or supplies. We have been offered large plastic stimulators and small rubber vibrators. 'Bring more money into the salon!' the postcards cry. Now that our local hairdressers' charges have gone up for the third time in two years, we are seriously thinking of trying it out. We have for some some time been trimming the hair of our children with the rabbit clippers, and have acquired some small skill. In fact, last week we trimmed our rather shaggy cocker spaniel to perfection. It is only a question of changing over to bigger game, and we have offered, for half the official price, to cut the hair of our new graduate assistant in a salon we have established off the feed-room in the animal house.

Short Back and Sides

IT distresses me that I can no longer obtain an honest haircut, of the type to which I became accustomed as a small child in my native Scotland. I used to sit on a high stool in the barber's little shop, and as the presiding genius shook out the white towel ready for the next customer I would hand over the sixpence which had been tightly clutched in my perspiring hand; both parties to the transaction would be well pleased.

Nowadays Scotland is inadequately equipped with such places, and the shiny establishments I am forced to patronise are staffed exclusively by young women to whom the words 'short back and sides' convey absolutely nothing whatever. 'Is it a trim?' they ask doubtfully, and on having the instructions repeated, with accompanying gestures, they may turn nasty and ask if I want it tapered or shaped. Or do I, perhaps, require it styled? They then proceed, with the utmost delicacy, to snip 3.15 mm off the hanging baskets covering my ears, and a similar amount from the cascade descending from my external occipital protuberance. Nothing I can say or do will induce them to perform otherwise, and the look of hurt reproach on their innocent little faces precludes actual violence. So I flounce out to hand over my three quid with a heavy heart, for I know that a return visit will be called for in about ten days.

It was never like this in Pop Poullis' establishment in North Queensland, where my unit spent a couple of years of the war. Not for him the effete precision of scissors; he relied exclusively on a comb and an electric mower which he swept upwards over my scalp, destroying everything in its path. The operation was swiftly over, and my only complaint was that the pin-ups which festooned his walls were just out of focus when my antigas spectacles were removed.

Since then I have had my hair cut in many different surroundings in all four quadrants of the globe. Perhaps the most exciting maestro was an Italian expatriate in a lady's hairdressers palace in a suburb of Cleveland, Ohio, who insinuated me as a favour into the salon, and informed me that his last male patient had been Marshal Badoglio. There was also a sinister back-street joint in Papeete, and a place in New York where a pigeon, which had lately featured on television, was in residence among the bottles of hair lotion. But the romance of such occasions has gone, and my user satisfaction has declined to zero as financial ruin approaches.

However, one branch of hairdressing has remained true to its great tradition; the other day I took my cocker spaniel to the kennels to be professionally tidied up before the advent of visitors. He emerged closely shaven and looking like a champion; the cost of this splendid job was only four times that of my own haircuts, and he looks as though he will stay like this for at least a few months. At last I know where to go for my next haircut.

The Prosthesis

DURING the late hostilities an old friend of ours incurred the gratitude of an army dentist by inoculating him with a sharp needle. When our friend later developed an apical abscess in an upper incisor, the dentist dismantled the tooth with loving care and substituted an affair of wire and plastic, cunningly wrought by his own hand, and moored invisibly to the adjacent teeth. The substitute was stained with Naafi tobacco juice to match its neighbours, and the general effect was most pleasing. Later, when the moorings relaxed their grip somewhat, the tooth would vibrate agreeably in our friend's head during the purple passages of his lecture on hygiene. This tooth, which we may call the Mk.I prosthesis, had a chequered history, but was ultimately lost at the bottom of the Minch during a rough trip to Stornoway in a tank landing craft.

The Mk. II prosthesis was not obtained until after the war. This time the matter was attended to with due form and ceremony, steaming moulds and plaster casts, and our friend found himself with a large pink serrated job occluding the whole of his hard palate. At one corner of this massive contrivance, as if by accident, was attached a single tooth. Our friend viewed it with considerable distrust, the more so since it transpired that every taste bud he possessed was located in the occluded area. He was spared much anxiety, however, by the resourceful action of his wife, who trod on the prosthesis on the bathroom floor the night he brought it home and snapped off a good three-quarters of the pink part. This allowed some at least of the taste of dried egg to penetrate his dulled senses at breakfast. He was also fortunate enough to shut the prosthesis in a drawer shortly afterwards, breaking off another large portion, and thereby allowing both the prosthesis and his tongue to occupy his mouth at one and the same time. Nevertheless he remains incurably disposed to remove his tooth when anything worth tasting is to be tasted, and when sneezing he has to adopt a complicated manoeuvre with his tongue lest the prosthesis should be expelled among the startled bystanders.

Our friend has now taken to academic life, and the other day he was seated in his lab. chewing on a well-earned Blue Danish sandwich when the door suddenly opened and a minor procession arrived, headed by the Vice-Chancellor, who was on a tour of inspection of scientific plumbing arrangements. Our friend rose rapidly to his feet and looked hastily for his tooth; to his dismay he found it was not in its accustomed place on the typewriter. His muttered responses to Authority lacked conviction, but they served, and it was not until he pulled out his hand-kerchief to mop his brow that the situation was irretrievably lost. With the handkerchief came the Mk.II prosthesis, which arched through the air and fell with a thin clattering noise full at the feet of the entire Drainage Commission.

Breathing

A physiologist of our acquaintance went through a frightening experience the other night. Returning tired but happy from his daily battle with recalcitrant electrons, he found his wife lying flat on her back in the middle of the living-room floor with one hand on the upper reaches of her sternum and the other on the region of her pylorus. She was hyperventilating strongly, and there was an admiring audience of children on the sofa. The weather was fine and cloudless, the barometer was high, and the hour was 6.15.

Though a physiologist, our acquaintance has not forgotten how to take a case-history, and he shortly elicited the fact that his wife was Breathing, having found out at 5.59 from her guiding women's magazine that Breathing was Life and that Tenseness was caused by Shallow Ventilation. It also transpired that his wife had been Breathing Wrongly and Inefficiently all her life, and that he, a specialist in human function, had never observed this elementary fact; the least he could have done was to have taken the trouble to ascertain whether or not his dependants were Breathing Properly. It was no thanks to him that his children were not yet Tense and that his wife had not contracted Tuberculosis.

Our acquaintance could make but little of the situation, and was therefore glad when, after a few more minutes during which the curtains billowed and swayed in the violent air currents and the shade of the hanging light vibrated danger-ously, a knock was heard on the door. Conscious of her social obligations, his wife immediately scrambled up, and, having by this time a serious alkalaemia, fell flat on her nose, scattering the audience on the sofa and disrupting a large pink balloon, the property of the smallest spectator.

Our acquaintance had his supper without further comment.

Cash Withdrawal

HAS anyone done a time-and-motion study of the removal of pennies from a money-box? I do not mean one of those new fangled contraptions with lock and key, but a stern uncompromising money-box cast in stout metal, with no concessions to human frailty beyond a forbiddingly narrow slot. The withdrawal of large irregular objects through narrow and ill-adapted orifices is a familiar problem to the proctologist and obstetrician, but their orifices are to some extent dilatable, whereas the money-box slot is rigid enough to baffle even a neurosurgeon. In view of the lack of recent literature on what is, prima facie, a surgical emergency, I am offering the fruits of my own experience in one consecutive case.

The operator should lie in the Trendelenburg position holding the box upside-down over his chest. An E.N.T. surgeon's head-lamp is an advantage at this stage, for it enables the presenting part to be clearly visualised. Perhaps I should here disabuse the beginner of the idea that the viscus necessarily contains money. Its physiological contents are pennies, half-pennies, and farthings, but almost equally common are pathological inclusions such as trouser-buttons, dead matches, pieces of 'Plasticine', and torn up postcards. The presence of safety-pins usually indicates malignancy.

In the initial exploration, brisk succession will define the extent and probable duration of the operation. Indeed, it may bring on a brief overflow of incontinence, which must not be mistaken for evacuation of the viscus. If the operator is not to leave a residue of unknown nature and amount, the passage of an instrument is always necessary. The size of the slot is a limiting factor, but the blade of a kitchen knife is most generally suitable. This is manoeuvred inside the box, at first gently and then more vigorously, after the fashion of a leucotomy knife. In the present case half an hour's manipulation of this kind yielded 1s. 9¾d., with a standard deviation of ±1.5 trouser-buttons. The impulse to reach for a lithotrite or cranioclast when faced with such a return must be sternly resisted. On the other hand, a small magnet can be safely used to remove small ferruginous foreign bodies, such as coupling-hooks from a model train, which so often precipitate an acute retention.

A Journey North

DURING the recent unseasonable outburst of fine weather an adventurous colleague of ours penetrated as far as Scotland on his summer holiday. Owing to the mysterious workings of destiny, his wife—the Master Planner of such occasions—was absent on the Continent at the time the expedition set off, and our colleague found himself in sole material and moral charge of his car, his two small children, a cocker spaniel puppy, and the various adnexa appropriate to such company. Our colleague's younger child becomes notably queasy on car journeys, and under the driving-seat he keeps a quantity of assorted oily rags and handkerchief tissues, together with a small portable vomitorium which started life as a jelly-mould. In addition he exhibits a 'Kwell' before each trip of any length, with results that are sometimes gratifying.

The first day, our colleague tells us, went well. His children fought unobtrusively on the back seat to the accompaniment of ear-splitting shrieks, and the puppy attempted to commit suicide by struggling through the window in the intervals of strenuously licking the back of our colleague's neck at unexpected moments in the thick of the traffic. Toffee papers blew in our colleague's face, it rained so immoderately that he could scarcely see the back of the lorry in front, and he was stung by a wasp. In short, a perfectly normal drive.

The next morning, flushed with his easy victory of the day before, our colleague not only omitted to establish a satisfactory blood-level of hyoscine in advance of breakfast, but also unthinkingly permitted the consumption of bacon and eggs. It was not until he was tying the rope around the luggage on the back of the car that he was brought to his senses by his younger child intimating that she felt sick, Daddy. The situation was difficult but not insuperable. Hastily producing a Kwell, our colleague rammed it in and sent the children off on a run with the dog to shake it down. On their return he subjected his younger child to a brief clinical examination; her deportment and colour appeared within normal limits. It was getting late, and our colleague had three hundred miles to go.

They had gone twelve of them when the inevitable happened. Our colleague had been listening to the snatches of sacred song from the back and was congratulating himself on an undeserved escape when, in the middle of the second verse of Jesus bids us shine, the Kwell shot across the car like a bullet and embedded itself in the dashboard. Fortunately our colleague was not in the direct line of fire, and the brunt of the main attack was taken by the puppy, who set up a pained barking. With some difficulty our colleague manoeuvred the car to the side of the road and produced the handkerchief tissues and the oily rags, it being now too late for the small portable vomitorium. During the mopping-up operations it proved necessary to remove his younger child's new coat, which he laid carefully on a wall beside the road until he had serviced the underlying cardigan and dress. After he had cleaned up the car and pacified the spaniel he inserted another Kwell and started off again to the accompaniment of further sacred music. It was not until fifty miles further on that his younger child complained of feeling cold . . .

Passport Problems

MY wife and I are going on a trip abroad from which she must return before I do, and we have had our single passport converted into two. This was done by extending its availability and deleting my wife, who was given a brand-new shiny passport of her own. We now find, on inspecting the newly arrived documents, that my wife can go to the Canary Islands, Iceland, Madeira, or the Azores, and I cannot follow her. It is little consolation to know that we may visit Algeria or the United States in company, and that neither of us can go to Peru; nor does it soften the blow that I have a Foreign Secretary's autograph while she has none. Since the passports came I have noticed my wife thinking, and there is a gleam in her eye I do not like.

Father Christmas

RECENTLY an industrial consultant we know drew our attention to the fact that nobody has considered the occupational hazards incidental to the work of professional Father Christmasses—or should it be Fathers Christmas? 'Goodness knows,' said our friend, 'there has been enough literature on Father Christmas, but never a good solid medical investigation.' We were impressed by his earnestness, the more so as we had once encountered a Father Christmas with a black eye, and we determined to make some inquiries.

A chap who works all day in a grotto is of course just asking for it. Swathed around with cushions of hot uncomfortable padding, his feet in rubber boots, his respiration impeded by immense whiskers, coughed and whispered at by untold thousands of highly infective Little Ones, he might just as well ring up the Emergency Bed Service before he starts. We took along a thermometer to a local grotto the other day, and we made the temperature 81°F. We would have liked to take the temperature of the Father Christmas, too, but it would have cost us two shillings, so we let it go. The grotto was filled with Little Ones in dripping oilskins, and the relative humidity was at least 90%; we estimated that the atmosphere had already been used four times. Though the press of business prevented us from penetrating as far as the North Pole, where Father Christmas had set up his consulting-room, our assistant reported that he was 'awfully hoarse, Daddy, and coughing dreadfully.'

Then there is the psychiatric side. The wretched Father Christmas is required to make articulate and impressive conversation in response to these incomprehensible whispers or stolid adenoidal stares, knowing that all he has at his back is a hundred dozen boxes of blow-football at one and seven, and a similar number of post-office sets at one and fourpence halfpenny. The music is also highly traumatic. We know of a Father Christmas who, after the fifteen hundred and seventeenth performance of *Jingle Bells*, inserted a blow-football outfit into the fairy organ and with set jaw watched it grind to a halt halfway through the fifteen hundred and eighteenth.

All things considered, we believe it should be scheduled as a dangerous calling. When we have assembled our information we are going to write to *The Lancet* about it.

Spaceman

WE know a chap whose great ambition it is to take off as a Space Physiologist in the first manned rocket to leave for Mars.

His body is in the lab., where it efficiently deals with oxygen tensions and so forth, but his mind, like that of Walter Mitty, is continually pulling gleaming levers or repairing the starboard stabiliser (which has had an argument with a meteorite on the Jupiter run). We have tried to discourage the chap, for we are old Spacemen ourselves, from the days before Space became respectable and got into the Sunday newspapers. Our shelves groan with the accumulated works of H.G. Wells, Arthur C. Clarke, and Ray Bradbury, and we have on file the weekly adventures of Dan Dare, Space Pilot of the Future.

It is the fauna that we worry about chiefly. When Dare arrived recently on Phoebe we had hoped that the locals would turn out to be an improvement. Less *green*, if you know what we mean. While this is gratifyingly true, we still cannot regard them with equanimity. That curious infraorbital hypertrophy bodes no good, and the polychromatic pigmentation speaks of a respiratory mechanism based on copper. Where there is copper (or metal of any kind) there is trouble, and indeed half our misgivings as to our acquaintance's future in Space are based on the incurable rapacity of its denizens. Our petty Tellurian atomic squabbles are as nothing to the rows which develop elsewhere in our own small planetary system. What must go on in other systems we shudder to think.

We have put these points forcibly to this physiologist chap, but to no purpose. We think he is just rocket-conscious. It appears he never merely leaves for lunch, he 'blasts off', and while travelling in other people's cars he is prone to lean forward urgently and snap out 'Cut both!' in moments of emergency. It is quite clear to us that he will either explode or wind up as an asteroid, and all we can say is good luck to him.

Musical Expression

OUR youngest grandchild now has to put out his tongue in order to draw a picture properly, and this reminded us that we had a cousin whose mouth becomes contorted every time he cuts his toenails, and a nephew whose facial tic appears only when he is peeling potatoes. These phenomena recalled a study we made some time ago of the physical expression of emotion by musicians.

We used to enjoy playing the piano, but we soon realised that some solo instrumentalists plumb the depths of anguish. The pianists are either exhibitionists in the style of Pachmann, or inhibitionists of the school of Rachmaninoff and Horowitz. It is the first group who suffer. The raised eyebrows, the hunched shoulders, the closed eyes, the head bowed to the keyboard while one hand reaches to heaven and the other sustains a single note—all these bespeak an intense and widespread emotional discharge. The inhibitionist group, which includes other keyboard performers, such as harpsichordists, use no muscle in either face or limbs that is not absolutely essential to the matter in hand.

Violinists, who of necessity have part of their face and neck immobilised, tend merely to lurch up and down (sometimes alarmingly) in moments of stress. Solo cellists, under no such restraint, sometimes go into generalised facial and bodily convulsions. Oboists and clarinettists, handicapped by the need to blow, have to restrict their emotional outflow to the upper part of the face, though they can menace the four corners of the hall and the heavens above with their instruments. Brass soloists also express what they can with their foreheads, and in addition make full use of their sweat glands.

Emotional display by members of symphony and chamber orchestras is obviously strictly suppressed, perhaps as savouring of individualism, personality cultism, or even revisionism, but in pop groups the wildest movements are obligatory, particularly during vocalisation. Not only are faces savagely twisted at every mention of love or desertion, but violent and perseverative epileptiform spasms of body and limbs testify to excitation spreading to every motor system.

At the conclusion of our investigation we wondered whether the incidence of psychiatric disorder among exhibitionist musicians thwarted by the mechanics of their instruments might differ from that in those able to give free rein to their psyche. Accordingly, we drew our observations to the attention of a neuropsychiatrist chap we know, and he has begun by sketching out a hypothetical network of central pathways originating from the musical part of Broca's area and including the latest and most fashionable peptide mechanisms. He only needs another three colleagues to establish the system in eponymous immortality.

Family Vomiting

A geneticist friend of ours found himself in an interesting position. From his youth he has been aware that in the matter of vomiting he is not as other men. Not for him the cough, the retch, the beads of sweat, the partial tearing of the abdominal muscles. All he has to do is switch in some hypothalamic over-drive and *up* it all comes. His wife, it seems, is cast in more fragile clay, and vomits in a routine manner. They have two children, both as a rule possessed of cast-iron stomachs. Nevertheless, the boy has succumbed to various infections, and our friend has been interested to observe on these occasions that his vomiting follows the maternal pattern. It is with the girl, however, that the future rests. In earliest infancy she was a good regurgitator, but for the last two years nothing would induce her to vomit. The other day she obliged on the dining-room sofa, and our friend was delighted to recognise at once a kindred spirit. He is now chattering happily about fourth-generation siblings, and he has already reserved a little black square for himself at the head of the family tree to be published in *The Lancet* of A.D. 2052.

Name This Child

ONCE in our callow youth we undertook to teach surface anatomy to Art students, and were struck by the fact that the names of the female members of the class differed widely from those of the female medical students with whom we had been used to associate. Our friends had been Jean or Margaret, Dorothy or Mary, but here were Dee-Dee, Merome and Lorrel, Demetria and Davilia. After some thought we arrived at the conclusion that although destiny may shape our ends, we rough-hew them to some purpose at the baptismal font. To give a girl a name like Nari or Kirrily is to direct her firmly towards the arts rather than the sciences. We were therefore encouraged to pursue our enquiries in the realm of secondary education, and nowadays if anyone asks our advice we consult an analysis prepared twenty years ago by our youngest child after study of the Schoolgirls Library file in the boot cupboard. At our request she categorized a series of names (n = 88) as 'goodies', 'baddies', 'fatties', and 'brains' and experience has shown that the results afford a reliable basis for predicting character and behaviour while *in statu pupillari*.

The survey revealed more goodies (70.5%) than baddies (19.3%). The eight fatties and the single brain constituted a neutral group, neither malevolent nor particularly public-spirited. Nor was any individual name significantly associated with adiposity. Exotic names such as Jocelyn or Gelda were more likely to lead their owners to become prefects, and (deplorably) among these holders of high office there were more baddies than goodies (p < 0.05): the three monitors, on the other hand, were on the whole a good influence.

Eighteen (29.0%) of the goodies had names beginning with J or P, and if parents want their daughter to rescue the head-mistress' dog from drowning or prevent the old study block from being burned down (by a prefect, naturally) they cannot do better than christen her Pam, with Patsy, Janet and Jenny as runners-up. If, on the other hand, they set store on unortho-doxy, and would applaud their daughter for joining the raffish group of prefects who meet behind the gymnasium for a quick drag and a bottle of crème de menthe, they should consider names such as Olga or Berril. Helen is a special case; three Helens in the series were solid upright citizens, but a fourth became a prefect and promptly (and perhaps inevitably) went to the bad. Parents have to be warned that the danger of this happening to a Helen is by no means negligible.

Those who wish their daughter to become brainy are re-grettably restricted in their choice, Viviane being the only certainty. And those who hanker after trendiness must select Sarah or Clare, the current favourites among top people notified in *The Times*. How these two will get on at school is nobody's guess, for they do not feature in the Schoolgirls Library data.

Visitors

OUR overseas visitors fall naturally into three groups. The first, composed of assorted relatives and friends, cause little trouble. They rarely venture outside, and simply sit in front of the fire, swathed in rugs, acidly expressing their amazement that anyone apparently in their senses should choose to live in this ghastly climate.

The second group are also fairly innocuous. These are the keen scientific types whose only ambition is to see the department and to discuss at inordinate length matters (often incomprehensible) of supposed mutual professional interest. They may consent to being taken for a drive round the district, but the conversation is usually strictly related to research and not to their current surroundings. Showpiece waterfalls and scenic mountain backdrops, moated granges and picturesque country pubs pass either unnoticed or unremarked. Their stay is brief, as they have to cover another twenty-six departments before taking off for another country on their study leave circuit.

It is the third group that cause alarm and despondency. They are also on study leave, but their inspection of the department and their academic conversation are relatively perfunctory. In contrast, their curiosity about everyday matters is intense, and an unending *feu de joie* of penetrating questions puts us to shame. 'Why is ITV not called Channel 3?' 'What is that yellow thing in the herbaceous border?' 'What are the differences between an English and an Irish setter?

In the car every shot in the fusillade lands with deadly accuracy outside our normal frame of reference. 'What breed are those cattle over there?' 'What do you call these lovely shady trees?' 'When does the salmon fishing begin?' 'Who lives in that big house?'

After a week of this our nerve cracks and we begin to answer at random; fortunately it does not seem to matter very much. But we are glad that our shattered confidence is relatively easy to rehabilitate. We go on study leave ourselves next year, and are accumulating a set of questions of our own.

Father's Examinations

IN our house we all walk very warily when Father brings home his exam books to correct. We can't have the T.V. on because it distracts him, we can't play the piano; we can't even talk to each other in whispers because he says nothing is worse than whispering. He sits at the dining table with a great pile of books and a succession of cups of coffee. Sometimes he gets so angry that he bangs the table with his fist and upsets the coffee cup, and sometimes he makes a funny sort of noise, and says 'Listen to this'. We all have to sit up straight and listen. When he says 'God knows I *told* them', Mother has to say 'Yes, dear', and when he says: 'How can morons like that hope to become doctors?' she has to say 'I'm sure I don't know, dear'.

Sometimes he has to get up and walk round the room, with his face very white or very red: 'bels palsi', he says, spelling it out, 'small ''b'', mind you!' and he puffs and blows and swears to himself for minutes on end. He writes down the worst spelling mistakes and posts them up on a blackboard in the department, and we think this raises his blood pressure. He lies awake at night thinking about how terrible his students are, and in the morning, his eyes are red and staring. He gulps his food down and his tummy rumbles dreadfully.

We are thinking of writing to the Vice-Chancellor to ask if he could do anything to get Father off having to correct these papers, because we are sure it is very bad for him. Not only that, it is bad for us; we think the students are lucky because they only have a couple of papers and a viva to sit, but we have to put up with the exams for three weeks or more every year.

Income Tax

WHEN I die, it is not Calais which will be found written on my heart but Income Tax. I spent much of my working life overseas, in a country whose tax treaty with Britain is totally incomprehensible, even to those whose job it is to interpret it, whose tax year begins on a different date, and whose exchange rate against sterling oscillates violently. The consequent strain of producing tax returns in both countries, thousands of miles apart, has excavated deep engrams in my limbic system.

In addition, my old adversary, the Inspector of Foreign Dividends, who regularly demanded multiple revisions and explanations of my written word, used to remain incommunicado for periods of up to three years from the time he received them; he would then disgorge a wholly unexplained refund cheque, the amount of which bore no apparent relation to the data provided. It is therefore not surpising that in my old age I tend to dream of a financial lifestyle in which income tax would not figure.

I can at once discount my chances of winning the football pools and appearing on television with a glamorous starlet, holding a cheque 6 feet wide and 3 feet tall, for £761,938.92. The reason is that I cannot understand the entry forms. 'Full perms 8 from 11, giving 165 winning chances' is too much for my fading I.Q. and the only bit I fully comprehend is 'moisten and seal'.

Nor would I be much good at the tables. I don't know the rules of baccarat, and I fear my youthful experience of poker in the R.A.M.C. would scarcely serve against the stony-faced men conjured up by my imagination.

It may be that I am too pessimistic to be a gambler. Even when I complete the weekly crossword I do not send it in to win the £10 book token, for I can visualise quite clearly the other 897 solvers who will send in correct solutions. I can't be bothered with the horses and the dogs, and amateur adventures on the Stock Exchange, even after the Big Bang, have very little chance of escaping the eye of the tax inspectors.

I have been thinking of converting myself into an offshore trust in a tax haven, and am currently investigating Jersey and the Isle of Man, but this is even more complicated than the football pools.

Nevertheless, my problem may be well on the way to solution through no action of my own. Yesterday I had a statement from my publisher telling me that the royalties due to me this year amount to 0.26p. I take this to be the beginning of a gradual slide in my income down to levels where income tax will cease to be payable.

The Trippers

MANY years ago I visited Radio City Music Hall in New York, and became one of the very few people ever to see a Radio City Rockette trip and fall on her nose during a high-kicking routine (fortunately without lasting physical damage, though the mental trauma must have been considerable). I found the experience both interesting and instructive, and I looked forward to making further such observations.

After an age of waiting, one arrived recently. I live close to a Scottish salmon river, where the wildlife includes dippers, goosanders, red squirrels and red and roe deer. There are otters, and an osprey occasionally comes to fish. At the top of the glen there is a pair of golden eagles. But, although agreeable, these phenomena are peripheral. The centre of my attention has always been the fly fishermen, haughty and aloof, who come from South of the border to spend an expensive week in waders in the middle of the current. I never wavered in my confidence that one day I would see one of them slip on a weed-covered stone and fall headlong.

The moment, when it came, provided almost a carbon copy of the affair in New York. The cries of alarm, the flailing of the limbs, the loss of dignity, and the lack of serious injury were all according to pattern; I felt fulfilled. The victim stumbled out with his waders full of water and his mouth full of deplorable language; I have never seen a man so wet.

Unfortunately I had not reckoned with Nemesis, and there was a sequel. A few days later, returning from my weekly visit to the supermarket with a shopping bag in either hand, I tripped over a protruding flagstone and fell forwards in exactly the same attitude as my two examplars, breaking my spectacles, cracking a rib, and bursting a bag of tomatoes all over my sweater. Whether this was a judgment or not, my appetite for this sort of thing has been temporarily sated.

Dr. Who's Vacation

I come from a family of highly skilled worriers, and I have inherited the talent. In the past most of my worries have concerned my puny personal affairs, but now they have become submerged in a more cosmic apprehension, a fear for the future of the human race. It seems certain that Dr. Who is to be relieved of television duty for 18 months, and though this period of rustication may eventually improve his efficiency (the Tardis has been more than usually prone to malfunction recently, and could do with an extensive overhaul and refit in space-dock), the Doctor's adversaries will not fail to profit by his absence. The Daleks are undoubtedly regrouping already, and the Cybermen, despite their last setback, are still a potent force for evil. As for the Master, his hand is everywhere. Little in the way of protection can be expected from the other Timelords. Despite their lack of consideration for their peripatetic trouble-shooter, they have relied on him for so long that they would now be completely useless in the sort of emergency he is wont to confront.

I possess no disintegrator, nor do I have a laser gun, and the small print in my insurance policies tells me that neither my life nor my property is secured against damage by extraterrestrial agencies. In the circumstances I fear that the best I can do to save the world is to barricade myself in the bedroom and wait despairingly to hear the terrifying command outside the garden gate: Seek! Locate! Exterminate!

Number Cruncher

MANY years ago a friend of mine went to live in the wilds of Cheshire, and while walking round the village shortly after his arrival was accosted by a small boy who introduced himself as 'Geoffrey, the one with the T.V.'. Nowadays I feel that I ought to introduce myself to newcomers as 'the one without the home computer'.

Yet one way or another I have had some little experience of what might at a stretch be called computing. In the 1939 – 45 war it was for a time my duty to turn the handle of a dusty R.A.M.C. adding machine (school of Babbage), and later I graduated to an electrical Friden, which buzzed and clicked very satisfyingly when suitably stimulated. Indeed, I count it as one of the triumphs of an essentially non-mechanical career that when it went wrong I shared the responsibility of taking the machine apart and restoring it to its pristine vigour.

Back in a university department after the war a new world of flashing red lights and noiseless operation presented itself, and I enjoyed working out the accounts of the tea club. The high point of my career came when I graduated to the university computer, crouched in its aseptic temple and approached with suitable reverence via a cascade of white-coated acolytes. This last experience involved a temporary reversal of the sleep rhythm, for the only time the god could spare for my insignificant problems was in the middle of the night. After this I became quite nonchalant, and at the drop of a byte would summon up literature searches in distant libraries overseas, or work out my income tax on whatever keyboard happened to catch my eye.

When I retired I was presented with a battery-powered pocket calculator, armed at all points with formulae and trigonometrical stigmata. This was packed, along with most of the rest of my worldly goods, in a shipping container which unfortunately permitted the entry of water, so that, among much other damage, my golden handshake was ruined.

The inevitable withdrawal symptoms began with tremor and sleeplessness, and I was therefore grateful to find that during the recent festivities Santa Claus had deposited in my stocking a solar powered number-cruncher, eager to do my bidding. For a time I was restored almost to normal, but a new and desperate crisis has now arisen: my beautiful and efficient cruncher has run out of numbers to crunch. Already the formication in my legs has returned, and this morning I had an attack of the shakes. It is clear that I shall have to go through a detoxification programme, but I am doubtful whether this should be graduated or 'cold-turkey'. Perhaps other sufferers would like to form a self-help group.

Victorian Culture

I can never pass a bookshop without going in, and so when a new and upmarket specimen opened its doors the other day I made a tour of inspection. The carpets were thick, the atmosphere suitably hushed and reverential, and on the shelves was an immense array of paperbacks, many of them labelled 'Classics.'

For some reason it came to me that this was the turning point, the crossroads of my literary life. I must now put aside my science fiction and my P.G.Wodehouse, and take a desperate plunge into Great Literature. In the aftermath of this decision the lust for possession took over, and I bought nine of the self-styled classics, selecting only those which promised to be readable. The set ranged from Tolstoy through George Eliot to Hardy, and I seasoned the lump with the unfinished novels of Jane Austen and plugged a couple of gaps in my knowledge of Dickens.

On the whole I survived the experience of reading them reasonably well, though I found the early stories of Henry James insipid, and Charlotte Bronte's *Villette* ran, as Dorothy Parker said of Katharine Hepburn, the gamut of emotions from A to B. Worst of all was the book from which, with memories of Boris Karloff, I had hoped much—Mary Shelley's *Frankenstein*. I had bought it in the belief that I would at one stroke elevate both my mind and the hairs on the back of my neck, but in both ways it failed me. The Baron, like Sherlock Holmes and Dracula, has become a household world, which testifies to the strength of the concept. But what a namby-pamby creature Shelley's monster was! What hand-wringing introspection, what a lack of suspension of disbelief, what soggy bad writing! I wonder how many people who accept this book as a classic have actually read it. Indeed, I wonder what is the definition of a classic, and who is responsible for applying the label.

Now sated with Victorian Culture, I have arranged my purchases on the mantelpiece, so that visitors can marvel at my erudition and breadth of interest. I have sent *Frankenstein* to the jumble sale, and taken down my set of Beatrix Potter; *she* knew very well how to push a good story along.

Distress of an Editor

SOME time ago I served a three year sentence as editor of a specialist journal, and the experience has left lasting scars. The virtual impossibility of guessing what the authors were on about led me to concentrate instead on the easier task of proof-reading. Once acquired, the habit of looking for mistakes instead of meaning is difficult to shake off, and recently it has involved my auditory as well as my visual input; I now listen to television in a state of considerable apprehension, for who knows what I may hear?

I have long been anaesthetic to the sound of plural nouns with singular verbs in egghead programmes. The latest recruit to a long list appears to be the world 'bacteria', which has joined data, media, graffiti, criteria, algae, vertebrae, and many others. It does not worry me that factors are nowadays said to 'mitigate' against success, and even phrases like: 'It was them that did it' and 'between he and I' (delivered in impeccable B.B.C. accents) merely induce a short run of extrasystoles. The English language changes, and who am I to hold it back?

But for some reason (no doubt my analyst could explain it) the now almost universal use of 'may' instead of 'might' in inappropriate circumstances causes a full charge of adrenaline to enter my bloodstream. I have heard a survivor of an accident say 'I may have been killed'—surely the ultimate in statements of uncertainty. 'The firm may have failed because of these debts' carries (for me) the clear implication that it has folded up, but the next sentence makes it clear that it is still in business, and the debts which *might* have been its downfall were actually paid off. Examples of this sort of thing occur daily, alarming my hiatus hernia and precipitating a variety of psychosomatic crises.

My most worrying recent experience occurred in the great world beyond the television screen. The girl in the local supermarket mistakenly punched up one of my purchases twice, and since the machine had no minus key she tried mentally to subtract 14p from the price of the next item, which was 46p. After some four suspenseful seconds of effort she called to a colleague: 'What's 14 away from 46?' Several more seconds passed. Eventually the other girl said: 'It might be 33'. Even the fact that she knew the word 'might' has failed to reconcile me to this conversation.

Bequest to Posterity

I well remember the day I first suggested to my family that I might write an autobiography. We were all at lunch, it was a fine sunny afternoon, and everything was peaceful, except for the cocker spaniel trying to get at the chops.

The first reaction was expectant smiles: what would the punch line be? But when it became apparent that there was no punch line, that I was in earnest, and actually intended to do this dreadful thing, their eyes widened, their pupils dilated, and one after the other they stopped in mid-chew. It was my son who first found words. 'But *you're* not famous!' he said, crystallising the general view of the gathering.

This was a shrewd thrust. I cannot conceal from myself that in the 20th-century hall of fame I cut no sort of figure. I did not discover penicillin. I was not under the table at the Yalta conference. I have never reached the Top Twenty or captained England, and I cannot claim to be the illegitimate son of Hitler's chambermaid. For autobiographical purposes these are grave disabilities. But just as Daisy Ashford's Mr. Salteena could not help not being quite a gentleman, I cannot help not being famous, and I said so, adding that I didn't see why only famous people should have the fun of writing autobiographies.

This did little to calm my dependants. Slowly their jaws began to move again, but above each head I could sense a small invisible bubble containing the invisible words 'God help us all!' They glanced cautiously sideways at each other to indicate how sad it all was, and the subject was tactfully changed.

For days afterwards I encountered little groups of people on the stairs or in the kitchen, usually attended by a worried-looking dog—people engaged in low-voiced conversations which broke up the moment I appeared. It seems that the main pre-occupation had now become the intimate revelations that such an autobiography might contain. If I was really determined on this desperate course, where would it all end? They knew their P.G. Wodehouse, and my activities had at once been equated with those of the Hon. Galahad Threepwood. The disreputable stories of family and friends, the law-suits, the blush-making sharing with strangers of matters best kept firmly concealed—all this was cause enough for concern. But perhaps I might eventually forget about it.

I did not forget. But after approaches to some 20 publishers – most of whom did not even examine my masterpiece – it became clear that it was destined, like so many exotic literary flowers, to blush unseen in my filing cabinet until a more discerning future generation takes over. If I had been a mass murderer, now, or a homosexual politician! But I fear it is too late to change my career in this direction, and I am resigned to my pitiful lack, not only of fame, but also of notoriety.

Weathermen

IN the city people pass each other in the street with no attempt at communication. But in this little Scottish town smiles are the rule, even from total strangers, and each encounter is embellished with verbal evidence of goodwill. A few of these are routine greetings, such as 'Hallo' or 'Good morning', which merely ask for reciprocation in kind, but most summarise the current state of the weather. Unlike the well-established responses of liturgy, replies to this kind of thing do not appear to have been codified.

'Lovely day!' cry the ebullient English holiday-makers when the sun is shining. 'Lovely morning!' exclaim the more cautious Scots, since who knows what an irritable Jehovah might not send us in the afternoon. The local Calvinists are even less enthusiastic and, after grudgingly acknowledging the sunshine, may add gloomily, 'We shall suffer for this later on,' or, if the temperature exceeds 15°C, 'Can't be healthy!' Bad weather provides a wider range of insights. Today the postman said to me, 'A bittie duller the day'—it was already raining heavily—and another chap, rather more terse, said merely, 'Colder'. This is a common gambit and usually correct. But a third man told me how nice it was that it had turned warmer, and a fourth, passing me while I was sheltering from the now pouring rain, said, 'Stormy kind!'

What are the appropriate answers to such judgments, which are phrased as statements but clearly require a brilliant and witty riposte? Up to now I have replied lamely, 'Yes, isn't it!', which is both unenterprising and cowardly. Yet to venture a modifying comment or disagreement is to invite discussion, and I must get home in time for lunch. Particularly troublesome are people who have programmed their speech centres according to a delusional climatic construct. 'Grand growing weather!' I heard somebody say without a hint of sarcasm one afternoon in

June when the temperature had failed to rise above 5°C and a force 7 northerly gale was bringing horizonal showers of sleet. Weakly to agree in such circumstances would betray my professional integrity, but to return a truthful 'No, it isn't!' would be an unthinkable rebuff to friendliness. I have decided in future to restrict my meteorological responses to a warm smile and wave of the hand, conveying no hint of a value judgment.

Transporter Phobia

GLANCING through the list of phobias in our medical dictionary the other evening we were struck by the absence of any mention of getting stuck on transporter bridges. We have never actually stuck on one ourselves, but we have always had an uneasy feeling that some day we might, and every time we drive on to the little platform high above the water we glance up at the fragile cables suspending us from the trolley rails and experience a dilution of our well-being. We are thinking, you see, that if the winding mechanism were to jam, the platform would stick half-way across. Our trips on transporters are invariably undertaken in a high wind, and we have no doubt that the stationary platform would soon begin to sway alarmingly above the chilly grey water. We have spent enough time in aircraft and landing-barges to realise that swaying platforms are no place for us, and besides we reflect that the van behind us might have defective brakes and suddenly precipitate us through the guard-rail. Or the cables might snap with a melodious twang. And so on: we are thoroughly cowardly about the whole thing. But it was only yesterday that we discovered a new and unsuspected risk attached to the journey. A biochemical friend of ours informed us with pride that he had actually stuck recently on a transporter, and we eagerly pressed him for details. (In addition to our phobia, we have a masochistic streak.) Yes, he said, the wind was high, the water perhaps rather colder than usual for the time of year. But it was not these considerations which moved him. As he drove on he observed that close alongside his port bow was an enormous lorry labelled at all points with slogans: DANGER; CORROSIVE; SULPHURIC ACID. It was after the second stoppage, when the platform had started to swing a bit—just as we thought—that our friend began to speculate idly as to the likely outcome if his car and the lorry should hit the water simultaneously. After the fourth or fifth halt he dragged his eyes away with an effort, only to notice for the first time another gigantic vehicle on his starboard beam, this time labelled DANGER; CORROSIVE; CAUSTIC SODA. Though a biochemist, our friend has not wholly lost touch with his inorganic training, and it did not take him long to work out that the contents of the two lorries would cause quite a reaction if mixed. By the seventh or eighth stop he had the equation straight in his mind, and got out of his car, determined to sell his life dearly. However, after the tally of stoppages had mounted to nineteen—it is a tribute to our friend's scientific spirit that he kept count—the transporter eventually berthed at the other side, and our friend drove off, disrupting the guard-rail and scattering foot-passengers right and left.

As far as we are concerned, this clinches the matter: we are not transporter-minded. When we looked in the mirror after our friend had gone we found two new white hairs.

Lighthouse Blues

IN our early youth we were sick on the second storey of the Eiffel Tower, and since this incident we have had little taste for heights. It is difficult to persuade us to enter an aircraft or even to paint the dining room ceiling, and on our seaside holidays we are a skeleton at the feast. While our dependants skip gaily along the smugglers' path, dislodging loose stones into the gulf 300 feet below, we are to be found progressing carefully on hands and knees, gripping the landward vegetation in an ecstasy of spasticity.

We were therefore disturbed to find, during our last summer holiday, that family opinion had committed us to visiting a lighthouse. Our confidence in the outcome was not enhanced after we had battered our way in a fifty knot wind to the foot of the structure and discovered that we were expected to sign away our chances of survival in advance. 'I the undersigned', said the form sombrely, 'hereby acknowledge agree and undertake for myself and for and on behalf of all minors noted hereunder as under my sole charge that no action suit claim or demand shall lie or be made or instituted in respect of any accident death injury loss or damage sustained or occurring by or to us or to any of us during the said visit. I will indemnify', went on the form, clinching the matter, 'keep indemnified and save harmless all departmental servants officers and agents against all actions suits claims and demands . . . .'

The lighthouse keeper was sleeping, and his assistant was seeing a man about a wreck, but trustingly permitted us to make the ascent unaccompanied. The minors under our sole charge occupied themselves happily in counting the 329 steps, and no accident death injury loss or damage was sustained or occurred on the way up. In the lantern room, however, the rarefied air and the presence of several other minors had the worst possible effect. Within seconds the lens holder, bearing the legend ON NO ACCOUNT TOUCH THE LENS HOLDER, had been seized and was rotating madly on its axis to the accompaniment of wild cries of exaltation. A dissipated-looking minor of a reflective turn of mind had begun to try to drop marbles on the head of the assistant keeper, and a smaller ginger group was running at high speed round the outside gallery, restrained from falling into the immeasurable depths only by a single rail at chest height. After one vertiginous glance through the open door we were forced to concentrate on the lighthouse keeper's box of dyspepsia tablets under the map of the local rocks and reefs. While we were thus engaged, the door to the outside gallery slammed and locked itself, and the minors under our sole charge, happening to be on the wrong side at the crucial moment, set up a prolonged bawling. With set and pallid face we descended the steps to fetch the assistant keeper with a key.

When order had been restored and we had indemnified and saved harmless the assistant keeper, we reached the ground again in an atmosphere of mutual congratulation. Only too soon a rough count established the fact that our personal quota of minors had been reduced by one. Elected a search party by popular acclaim, we climbed the 329 steps for the third time, to find our youngest minor flat on her stomach in the lantern room, deeply immersed in the lighthouse keeper's True Love Stories and sampling his dyspepsia tablets.

For our next holiday we are going to the Cotswolds.

Unhandyman

SHORTLY after we set up house in Western Australia my wife noticed some sinister black spots on the leaves of the umbrella tree which screened our dining room from the road. We might well have fallen into a nerveless panic, for the sum of our joint knowledge on diseases of umbrella trees is not as great as we might sometimes wish it to be. But a few months previously we had happened to make the acquaintance of a most erudite fellow countryman in the local nursery—a man who had been in Australia for forty years, and was reputed even to be able to distinguish a gum tree from a eucalypt. Our course of action was therefore clear, and we bundled the children, the dog, and two of the affected leaves into the car and set off for a consultation.

True to form, the oracle took less than two seconds to make the diagnosis, and indeed he did not have to let go the handles of his wheelbarrow. 'Smut', he said briefly 'it must be near an oleander'. A virtuoso performance like this always leaves me breathless, and, as usual on such occasions, I became a trifle flustered and unable to listen as accurately as might be to the details of the remedy. It appeared, however, that the tree should be sprayed with white oil, and we gratefully rounded up our entourage and set off for home, calling in on our way at the nearest hardware store.

Had I been less confused, this was a step I should never have taken, for I can never cross the threshold of a strange hardware store without a preliminary sinking sensation. These chaps behind the counter terrify me. Not only are they thoroughly schooled in the comparative merits of various sealers, primers and undercoats, they can discourse with equal facility on caulking materials, mowing machines, washing lines, and self-tapping screws; they can remember the sizes of hacksaw blades, and can actually understand the classification of sandpaper. In nearly every case this intellectual superiority is matched by a ferocious skill in dialectic. With a few merciless questions they can make public the fact that you are an incapable European, who has never been able to do anything for himself in his life—anything useful, that is, like building a boat, adding a new bedroom, or sinking a well. However simple your needs, in the way you ask for them there will be a fatal flaw which will expose you to ignominy. One crucial point will inevitably escape your vigilance, and this is the one upon which they will fasten, worrying the last drop of juice out of it until you are glad to admit total defeat and accept humbly whatever they choose to give you instead of what you originally thought you wanted.

There is only one way to avoid this sort of thing, and that is to confine your custom to one particular dispenser of hardware. I always choose the most genial and benign-appearing one in the district, having spent several days scouting around beforehand. On the occasion of my first visit I draw him aside and make a full confession of my essential uselessness, appealing to his basic humanity and throwing myself on his mercy. This approach is often quite successful, and we may even enter into a sort of tolerant patron-apprentice relationship, so that I am allowed to come into the shop and ask for things in low tones, out of earshot from the other customers.

In a strange hardware store, of course, this painstakingly established atmosphere does not exist, and I have to take my chance in the ordinary rough and tumble of commerce. Matters are not improved by the fact that when I come in there is always one of these unnerving conversations going on between the chap behind the counter and a local expert. You know the sort of thing:

'Got half a dozen twenties, Kev?'
'What d'you want 'em for, Fred?'
'Revetting the top four-by-twos' (That's what it *sounds* like)
'Is she turned yet?'
'No'
'Better with twenty-fours, then; give you a better purchase'
'But then you'd have to bed her in sideways, Kev, and there's no tolerance for the crosspieces'
'Couldn't you tom them up?'
'No, she wouldn't take it, you see, because of the bonding'
'Right then, Fred, twenties. What else?'
'Couple of dozen duplex brass ends'

And so it proceeds, at once impressive and totally incomprehensible, the communication of twin souls. How different are my own conversations:

'I want some white oil, please'

'Raw, or treated?'

(You see? At once the unexpected shaft, the one thing you never thought you would have to know. How the devil do you treat white oil? And why? For that matter, what on earth *is* white oil?)

'What have you got?'

(This gets nowhere; you know he must have both, but it may gain time)

'We can give you both'

'I'll have some raw oil then'

(After all it is a fifty-fifty chance, and raw is probably cheaper)

'How much do you want?'

'Oh, just a small bottle'

(Should be fairly safe; we can get more later)

'It doesn't come in bottles, only cans'

(The chap has already sized the situation up: here is a customer whose previous experience doesn't include buying white oil; almost certainly some useless egghead)

'Well, a small can, then'

'Three and a half, or seven?'

(Is this pounds weight, or fluid ounces? Or even pints? And why such peculiar sizes?)

'Three and a half will do, to try it'

(A fatal slip; the chap has been working up to this point: here comes the death blow)

'What exactly did you want it *for*, sir?'

The inclusion of the word 'sir' is an expression of the ultimate in contempt; the intonation is impossible to capture on paper. I have no alternative but to break down and confess that we want to spray an umbrella tree infected with smut by an oleander in the front garden. (How silly it all sounds when it is dragged out of me like this!) At once the chap's whole demeanour alters; he has crushed my resistance and he can now start to sell me something.

'You don't want white oil, sir, you want our special solution for smut. Made for us on the prescription of the Government analyst . . . carefully selected materials . . . full instructions on the bottle . . . and that'll be a dollar fifty. Thank you very much sir; if you have any more trouble come back and let me know.'

As I leave the shop I notice out of the corner of my eye that he has turned aside from the counter to spit.

Ever since my early youth in Scotland it has always been like this. If I ask for putty it is never the right sort, and my wretched requirements are dissected in ringing tones for everyone in the shop to hear. If I ask for a pound of nails they sell them by the dozen, and if I ask for a gross they sell them by the pound. It is almost worse if I write out a specification before I go in, for I have to read it aloud while the chap stares contemptuously above my head at a fly on the ceiling. A request for electric drill bits, based on an advertisement I saw in the morning paper and presented in this manner led to a public brainwashing which lasted fully eleven minutes before I collapsed. Even if all I am after is a few screws, I am certain to ask for a length which isn't made, or not to know whether they should be dipped or plated. Such interviews always wind up with the other customers waiting at the counter looking at each other silently, their lips curling. Doesn't the fellow *know* what he wants?

And even when I come home bearing my pitiful little parcel my troubles are not over. My wife has a yardstick for assessing the value of any husband of her acquaintance; if he has put up some shelves for his wife he must be all right; if he hasn't, his suitability as a husband is still in question. In our household the matter is still, after twenty-eight years, in doubt. First of all we didn't need shelves, because we shared a big rambling house that was well provided, and subsequently we occupied houses where there was no room for a shelf. But the matter is only temporarily (forgive me) shelved, and there is no doubt that at some future time I must undergo my aptitude test for matrimony. It is futile to attempt to lay in the scales the Venetian blinds repaired, the ceiling painted, the bathroom tiled, the linoleum laid: the shibboleth is a shelf, and no substitute is acceptable.

Now I am not much of a hand with wood. Venetian blinds, yes; shelves, no. Even chopping firewood is not a simple matter for me. The anaemic sort of stuff I used to chop in Britain to keep the home fires burning gives but little and sorry practice for the chopping of jarrah. I bought a seven and a half pound axe (more ruthless exposures in the shop where I got it), and eventually managed to control it instead of it controlling me; even so, I still mis-hit occasionally and virtually paralyse both arms.

When it comes to the garden, I have never pretended to any expertise; I dig where I am told to dig, and when I am exhausted I cease digging. But for some reason my activities aroused immense interest in the minds of the next-door neighbours, who were keen to educate me in the local conditions. 'If you make it as deep as that', they said impressively, 'the rain'll never stay in it; they'll die in a couple of weeks.' The family across the road were also eager to help the new chum. 'You'll have to have it much deeper than you've got it now, or else their roots won't be able to breathe.' After a Saturday afternoon devoted to this sort of thing I have to lie down most of Sunday. I think they all thought I would soon catch on; after all, I hadn't been educated properly over there, but that wasn't my fault.

But as time goes on and I still haven't tiled the roof, rebuilt my radiogram, dug and poured a swimming pool in the back yard, renewed the guttering or relined my own brakes, it is gradually being borne in on them that I am only a second-rate citizen, to be tolerated, perhaps, but certainly not worthy of having time wasted on me. After all, I don't even have a proper workshop built on to the house (with my own hands, naturally). I can't sail a fourteen footer, I can't make a surfboard. In fact, I am pretty much a dead loss.

A chap ought to be able to do *something*.

Microcomputer

MY son has gone on holiday, and has left his microcomputer in my charge, with strict instructions about what to rescue first should my house show any tendency to burn down. This sacred trust has allowed me to explore the personality of the computer, as well as its more mundane capabilities as an entertainer and instructor. Strangely, the personality varies markedly according to what it is doing.

When it plays Scrabble, it is a model of gentlemanly sportsmanship. In the delightful interchange preceding the actual game it is at pains to ascertain my name and to make me thoroughly at home as we settle together the details of the coming encounter. During play it betrays no sign of animosity, apart from dealing me out improbable combinations of letters such as QJKIIOO. When, in desperation I enter a word such as THRIIW, its challenge is couched in the mildest of terms: – 'Are you *sure* about THRIIW?' If, in a futile attempt to stave off defeat, I answer 'Yes', the computer bows to the superior knowledge of a native English speaker, and replies 'Word accepted'. Nothing could be more civil.

But when I attempt to write programs, all geniality disappears, and communications are confined to cold and terse comments such as 'Variable not found', 'Nonsense', or 'Statement lost'. Any attempt to answer back in kind is futile, for it holds the whip hand. And when I try to use it as a word processor, communication is replaced either by dumb insolence or by active interference. The cursor disappears, valuable sentences are lost, and paragraphs shift wildly up or down, but always to the wrong place.

Worst of all, at chess the computer, which at first appears grave and responsible, soon displays the baser side of its nature, for it cannot bear to lose. Immediately an unexpected move is made (most of my moves are unexpected, even by me), it begins to sulk, and may arbitrarily denounce it as 'invalid'. If it finds itself so hard pressed that disaster looms ahead, its usual response is to shut itself off and refuse to continue playing, but yesterday I caught it out in more forthright cheating. It had been unwise enough to allow my queen to fork its king and a rook, and this sent it into silent but doubtless bitter self-recrimination lasting for eight minutes. Then, quite brazenly, in front of my eyes, it converted my white queen into a black one, leaving two black queens on the board. Only then did it shut down all possibility of further communication.

My stewardship is nearly over, and I shall find it difficult to make the transition from the Computing mode to my more usual Housekeeping mode, from pixels to fish fingers, from FOR NEXT loops and GOSUBs to corn flakes and frozen peas, from BINs to dusters, and from POKEs, PEEKs and STRINGs to silver polish and the laundry. But although I shall miss our cosy games of Scrabble, on the whole I have found the computer to be user-inimical, and I shall be delighted to hand the wretched thing back.

Early Warning

WE are daily assailed by warnings that the population is ageing, and that in 40 years a handful of wage-earners will be attempting to support a ponderous agglomeration of unproductive and senile citizens. A colleague recently pointed out to us that attention has not been adequately drawn to the increase in the rate of advance of old age and adduces as evidence the fact that for him the millennium is here and now. Though a man of only some 38 winters, his ulcer is already well established, and his asthma and rheumatism trouble him at night. His discs do not prolapse in a well-conducted way, but moulder away quietly, and already he has reached a stage of forgetfulness which would do credit to a stage professor. The crowning blow came the other day, when he went to his dentist for a regular check-up and was told that his teeth were being attacked by a disease of old age.

Unfortunately the potential wage-earners in his family are not yet of an age at which he can hand on the torch to them, being 6 and 2 respectively, so he is battling on despite his manifestly outworn mental and physical equipment—a man in advance of his time.

The Mysterious Movies

IN my youth, when all my wits were still in working order, I was an enthusiastic cinema-goer. In those far-off days of silent pictures you could tell the baddies from the goodies by their black hats and their evil sneers when they thought nobody was looking, and little cerebration was necessary to divine the general outline of the plot. Even when, with the coming of sound, dialogue became an important factor, my razor-like brain could usually cut to the heart of what was going on without assistance.

The rot began in 1946, with the release of *The Big Sleep*, which I could not understand at all (I gather that the author and the director were not very sure what it was about either), and matters gradually became more and more complicated, particularly in respect of thrillers. Now, when I visit the cinema to see one, I have to take with me a minder to explain things.

My upper register hearing is not what it once was, particularly in a half-empty cinema where the sound bounces off the walls, and it takes me some minutes to get accustomed to rapid and confidential speech in strong regional accents or dialect. During this time I often miss vital background exposition.

Why were the diamonds in the desk and not in the safe? How did they know that the courier would be murdered? Who are all these women? Many such matters can subsequently be sorted out over a cup of tea and a biscuit with my minder, but if only the directors would refrain from plunging into the action before my cerebral decoding system is ready for it, postmortems of this kind would be unnecessary.

Now that my nearest cinema is thirty miles away I have less opportunity to indulge my feeling for the medium. However, on a recent holiday of three months in Australia, where filmgoing is still accorded a proper respect, I managed to chalk up 19 new titles, several of them not yet released in London, and at least 3 of them were perfectly comprehensible.

Highland Games

UP here our microclimate has escaped from the control of the Weather Centre, and orders its own affairs. A television forecast of 'sunny periods' now guarantees a day of 10/10ths sullen grey cover, and 'a few clouds developing by evening' translates as 'a persistent downpour beginning at dawn and lasting all day'.

It was therefore a shock to find that our annual Highland Games fell on a decent day—the only one we had had in the past eight weeks. The sun shone on the bulging muscles of the heavies, on the lassies dancing nimbly on a strangely dry platform, and on the pipers who rang the unexpectedly visible welkin. After the concluding ceremony the mobile bank and the Army recruiting van drove away unassisted, instead of having to be winched out to safety, as had been universally predicted.

All this was very satisfying, but I had another reason for contentment, for my grandchildren were otherwise occupied, and in consequence I was spared the annual loss of face which attends my refusal to take a ride in any of the giant mechanisms—Rotors, Octopuses, Racers, and the like—which lurk among the sideshows.

When I was a boy I roller-coasted with the best, but advancing years took toll on the cells in my vestibular apparatus, and I came to realise that thrills of the kind that my dependants would have me sample are not worth the aftermath. My family image began to disintegrate because I would not embark on the scenic railway in the Tivoli Gardens in Copenhagen, and for many years thereafter my negative attitude (maintained against frightful odds) was an inexhaustible source of adverse comment. The matter was finally settled in Disneyland, where, despite minatory notices about people with heart conditions or nervous dispositions, I was dared by my daughter to enter the Magic Mountain, in which sensory deprivation and fearsome G-forces induced in me both pity and terror. The resultant vertigo put me out of action for two days, and since then it has been accepted by the F1 generation that poor old Dad isn't fit for this sort of thing. This viewpoint has unfortunately proved difficult to instil into the F2 generation, and it is pretty universally felt that Grandpa is something of a fraidie-cat.

But this year at the Games there were no reproaches. I was able to remain upright throughout the day, and enjoyed the calmer and less adventurous attractions. No doubt next year will again bring the usual ruthless criticisms of my inadequacy.

Lack of Recognition

IN our recently acquired role as absent-minded senior citizen we seem to attract a certain amount of obloquy. The other day a young lady charged us publicly with snootiness because we had stared blankly through her as she passed us in her car.

We have never been good at faces, and when they are concealed in the dim twilight behind a steamy windscreen advancing at 30 or 40 m.p.h. our record is admittedly abysmal. Nor do the cars themselves help us. Our grandchildren can instantly name and give the full specifications of anything on four wheels at a distance of two hundred metres, but we cannot even distinguish one moving carapace from another, and this prevents us from deducing the identity of the white blotch or blotches inside.

Indeed, we have always regarded cars mainly as possible agents of our personal destruction, and tend to limit our apprehensive gaze to the bonnet, which we reckon is the bit that will hit us first. We are thus little better informed than the Latinist Godley when he wrote:

'What is this that roareth thus?
Can it be a Motor Bus?
Yes, the smell and hideous hum
Indicat Motorem Bum.'

In the days when we were charged with the instruction of preclinical students we used to be quite unable to recognize them when we met them again at the final year dinner, for most of the males who once had whiskers had by then shaved them off, and most of those who had been clean-shaven now sported consultant-type beards. As for the females, a different hair-style was always enough to short-circuit our memory banks.

Now, when we have to deal with a restricted number of bank tellers and check-out girls instead of a multitude of students, it might be expected that matters would improve, but a change of milieu and dress is just as off-putting as ever it was, and when out for a Sunday walk we have often engaged in spirited conversation with people who look vaguely familiar at the time, but only click into place hours later as the girl in the fish-shop or the local librarian.

Matters came to a head yesterday, when outside the supermarket we failed to recognize and respond appropriately to the hostess of a party we had attended the night before; she had unsportingly equipped herself with a hooded anorak and a strange dog belonging to a friend.

We have come to the conclusion that it is less traumatic to stay at home and watch the telly.

Golden Jubilee

I QUALIFIED in medicine in June, 1937, so that I have now entered my 50th year as a doctor. As a result all the doubts I have had in the past regarding jubilees and centenaries have been revived. The Festival of Britain, intended to indicate the half-way mark of the 20th century, generated a considerable correspondence in *The Times*, and it was this that was originally responsible for my misgivings. The point at issue was whether the Festival should take place at the beginning of the year 1950 or at its end—whether the triumph was to have reached the 50th year or to have completed it without disaster. Inevitably this led to an argument about whether the century should be considered to have begun on Jan 1, 1900, or Jan 1, 1901, and this rather red herring shifted the debate to the date of the birth of Christ, a subject which I have no intention of bringing up here.

On the whole I still favour the school of thought which rested its case on the fact that no batsman is applauded for making a century until he has completed his hundredth run, and on this basis I ought not to celebrate until June 1987. This would be in line with the fears of my mother, a staunch Presbyterian, who would never allow me to have my birthday party even a day ahead of time, even if it was administratively highly desirable to do so. Her reason was that I might be struck down by a vengeful Jehovah for her arrogance in assuming that I would survive until the correct date.

But such considerations do not seem to worry the institutions —universities, medical schools, colleges, hospitals, and learned societies—with which I have been associated. Presumably, as corporate bodies, they consider themselves immune from divine retribution, for they arrange Jubilee Years preceding the actual anniversary, with congresses, commemorative dinners, honorary degrees, and, in pride of place, Jubilee (or Centenary) Building Appeals.

Having thought the matter over carefully, this is what I intend to do myself, notwithstanding the possibility of disaster. For my Jubilee Year I have already composed a Private Housing (Renovation and Amenities) Appeal, and I am now advertising for an Artist in Residence.

Final Stages

YOU can tell I am getting on a bit. When I was young, bus conductresses called me Dear or Love, and on a visit to Glasgow I was somewhat menacingly addressed as See you Jimmy. After I qualified, Doctor became my due, and as my teaching posts increased in seniority the use of Sir by students anxious to win friends and influence people was a source of gratification. Ultimately Prof became the watchword within the department (it was kept deadly secret during casual social encounters out-side, for nothing dries up a conversation more quickly than the knowledge that you are speaking to an untouchable). Nowadays Sir is used with distressing frequency by the general public, and specialists such as car-park attendants or motorists who wish to accuse me of wrongdoing call me Dad or Grandpa.

When I ask for directions in the hospital they are given very slowly and with emphasis, and are followed by a quiz to make sure they have penetrated the layers of fog surrounding my higher centres. And I am occasionally recognised by a student who claims I taught his grandfather before the war.

The check-out girls in the supermarket have started filling up my plastic bags for me very carefully, and counting out the change I produce from my pocket in front of my eyes so I can be quite certain what is happening. It is only a question of time before I shall feel the touch on my elbow heralding the approach of a senior citizen anxious to help me across the road.

Film Trapping

LAST week my nerve finally cracked and I bought a video-recorder – a step which had been urged upon me by my family and friends for years. I had resisted so long before joining the multitude because of my fears that there would be too many control buttons for me. The remote control of my television has 21 buttons, but their functions are reasonably obvious and they are labelled in what passes for English. The programmable control of my recorder has added another 34 buttons, most of which are identifed merely by cabalistic signs. Six of them, I am glad to say, appear to do nothing.

When I qualified in medicine I never envisaged a career as a button presser, and I have never been button-minded. But now, fifty years on, and after intensive study of the manual, my fingers play across the buttons like those of a latter-day Rubinstein, and I experience an awesome sense of power as the machine protestingly wakes to life to do my bidding.

I bought the recorder partly because of programme clashes, but also because of the ancient late-night movies, which I missed when they were new, and which have hitherto surged past my unheeding senses as I lay fast asleep.

I have in my time patronized a great variety of cinemas. There were first the smoke-filled picturehouses of my youth, redolent of coal-tar disinfectant, with the chap at the piano sketching the emotions I ought to be feeling at developments on the screen. Then came the more luxurious but equally smoke-filled establishments in London and elsewhere. It was not till I was posted to Australia during the war that I found that cinema-going could be divorced from cigarette smoking, and that it was feasible to have programmes shown at set times, with bookable tickets. The curse of continuous performances, with the screen intermittently blocked out by people clumsily entering and leaving at vital moments could thus be avoided.

For a time I was stationed in a small Queensland sugar town where the filmgoers sat on deck chairs under the stars; there were lonely singles and cuddly doubles all strung together on a series of metal poles. The moon rose hugely behind the screen, and great bomber shaped moths flickered in the light of the projector. As you sat, you might feel a mysterious heaving and struggling underneath, and if you investigated you might make contact with a wet nose, for the local dogs were movie fans and slept under the audience every night. In less ambitious places elsewhere I attended performances projected on the outside of a church hall or a barn.

My first encounter with a drive-in cinema was in Iowa City, where I was taken, after a hilarious party, to see Bob Hope through a slight haze of alcohol. My hosts organized Coke and foot-long hot dogs, and we had a marvellous time, only marred by the fact that we drove away with the speaker still inside the car; we were not popular with the management.

Since then I have sampled Cinerama, Cinemascope, 3D, Sensesurround and other phenomena in a great variety of buildings. But now the local cinema is my own flat, and instead of having to go out in the cold and wet to face parking problems and vandalism I can cause the films which formerly flashed through the darkness unseen and unheard to be ambushed and impounded by my vigilant recorder, so that *they* are forced to come and see *me* the next day.

Parting Shot

I began to shoot with a twelve-bore as soon as it was considered safe for me to do so. My father, a first-class shot, was a member of a syndicate which rented various grouse moors in Angus as well as some mixed shooting – pheasants, partridges, woodcock. In the syndicate most of the members were past middle age, and accordingly the head keeper of the shoot we had for several successive seasons docketed me in his mind as a 'fleet young b-----', and always gave me the task of climbing round the rigging of the hills as a flank gun with the line of beaters. It was hard work, and often the chances of a shot were few, but I was rewarded with some of the finest views in Britain. There were ptarmigan up there, and mountain hares, and a great stillness. The little burns sprang out from under my feet to tumble headlong through the stones and rough grass down to the heather and the river far below. The larks sang above my head, and in the far distance lay the striding line of butts, black against the purple hills.

I had less enthusiasm for standing in a butt waiting for driven birds. Yet there is much to be said for just waiting. If, as usual, I was at the end of the line, being considered fittest for the highest climb, I could often survey the whole situation, guns and beaters, and notice the progress of the drive. Here a too eager dog would allow a covey to slip out to the side well ahead of the man with the flag, whose curses would often be borne down on the wind; there a big hare would edge cannily between two of the lower butts, their occupants unconscious of its presence. We would eat together in front of the butts among the circle of dogs, each with his tongue dripping redly down the front of his chest. The bees worked among the heather, and occasional straying black-faced sheep came to stare angrily at the intruders.

On other occasions we went after capercailzie in a big wood on the edge of our shoot. When the beaters roused them off their chosen trees they left with a tremendous clatter, but then flew silently, like an owl, between the tree trunks and about six feet off the ground. The sudden appearance of a bird as large as a turkey, flying without a sound straight for your head, is an alarming experience, and I am not ashamed to say that the first time I ducked and did not even let off the gun. Some of the other places I shot over later on were isolated and wild; in another wood where there was a marshy place and a magnificent patch of blaeberries I saw a pine marten, and there were golden eagles in attendance, though I never knew where they nested. Buzzards came too, and the great hoodie crows, our enemies.

Besides having a share in the syndicate, my father used to rent a small shoot of his own, on the land round the sanatorium for which, as Medical Officer of Health, he was responsible. When we shot there we had to make an early start, so as to have a word with the local keepers before the rest of the party arrived. On such occasions our guns were taken out of their carrying cases about half past six in the morning, and loaded into the back of the car along with the cartridge bags and a couple of ecstatically shivering cocker spaniels, who were allowed to sniff the Rangoon oil to assure themselves that it was all actually true. By the time we had finished our breakfast the sky had begun to clear and the gaslight was yellow and faint; we set off in daylight on our fourteen mile run through the cold awakening countryside, the frost hard on the ground and often sparkling from every tree.

In the evenings we would come back in the dark, the rising moon shining in through the back of the car on the hessian sacks full of pheasants and hares; the dogs lay, totally exhausted and fast asleep, with their noses on top of the blissful smells inside the sacks. When we got home the bag was laid out by torchlight on the floor of the wash house, and a rough list was made for distribution to our friends – a brace of pheasants for one, a hare and a brace of partridges for another. Some were addicted to woodcock or to snipe, and these were always particularly remembered. We hung them up in bundles on the hooks in the rafters, and walked slowly in through the back door and along the kitchen passage, our faces burning with the cold wind, to clean and oil the guns. After a hot bath we settled ourselves for supper on a trolley in front of a blazing fire, and as likely as not it would be hare soup, dark and steaming, and roast pheasant, the spoils of our last expedition.

As a boy I had just as much enjoyment from rifle shooting as from my father's twelve-bore. At the sanatorium I learned to shoot rabbits with a rook rifle, and later, at school, when I found I took no pleasure in cricket, I happily transferred to shooting. The Dreghorn range, like everywhere else in Edinburgh, is a windy place, but my memories are of sunshine, the smell of rubber elbow pads fixed over my school blazer, the range telephone which was always out of order, and the mounting

excitement of seeing a series of large black discs raised to the
bottom right hand corner of the target, indicating a succession
of bulls. There was something peculiarly satisfying about the
details of rifle shooting, – allowing carefully for the erratic wind
and varying light, wrapping the sling round your elbow to
steady the complex formed by the rifle and your body, aligning
the blackened sights accurately, and squeezing the trigger so
gently that the shock of the recoil taken by your shoulder
muscles came almost as a surprise.

And even when you were not actually shooting there was
always the pleasure of marking – of sitting in line on the rough
benches under the corrugated iron roof of the five hundred yard
butts, hearing the whip and thump of the arriving bullets,
watching the kick and splutter of sand thrown up behind your
particular target and searching it for the neat round hole. Then
the exertion of changing the big targets on their iron frames, and
the lordly superiority of fixing the black marker in the hole,
lifting the target again, and signalling a magpie or an outer.
Sometimes there was even the thrill of waving the red flag (as
slowly as possible) from side to side to indicate a miss; if you
knew who was firing this waving might be prolonged indefinitely or until the telephone rang angrily.

I was too erratic to be much use at school, though I could rise
sometimes to an occasion. I went to Bisley with the school eight,
but had more successes with the clay pigeons and other
sidelines than on the thousand yard range. It was not until
much later that the high point of my rifle shooting career
arrived. For a time during the war I was medical officer to a
garrison town, and, like many such, was supremely bored with
routine. It was a delight to be offered the chance of testing some
rifles to be used for training purposes. There was plenty of
ammunition and I had a most pleasant colleague, a man who
had shot for South Africa not long ago. We developed a full
scale competition once we had sorted out the good rifles, with
a group at a hundred yards and competition scoring at two
hundred and five hundred. There was considerable barracking
during the occasion, and side bets were freely taken; it was
therefore very exciting when we found that we had both
obtained 'possibles' at two hundred, and had dropped one
point at five hundred. The crucial decider was therefore the
group, and when they were measured (by a financially involved

committee) mine was the smaller by half an inch. I tried to be off-hand about it, but failed.

Those were the only shots I fired during the war except for one magnificent gesture when, as a signal, I fired a service revolver into the air from a landing barge off the Great Barrier Reef. This is not the place to go into my motives, but it was a wonderful sensation. Now I come to think of it, I never cleaned that revolver.

I did not start to shoot again when I returned to Scotland, and the local pheasants and grouse have been safe from me for many years; my current cocker spaniel tyrant, who dictates my every action, would not know a hare from a roe deer. Indeed, his only contact with pheasants occurred when he fell through a crust of snow on top of one; it was difficult to tell which of the parties to the encounter was more surprised. The rifle and the gun were disposed of long ago, but they still act as a powerful focus for remembering the happiness of youth.

Bedtime

WE have just acquired a puppy of tender age, and he has been installed in a box in the kitchen. The first few nights we had him he cried like a baby and refused to be comforted until he was taken upstairs and allowed to crawl under the bedclothes of one of the junior members of the household. He wasn't cold, he wasn't hungry, he just wanted company in bed with him. But we did not receive an expensive physiological education for nothing, and we have rigged him up a heart-lung preparation in his box for him to sleep with. It consists of a rubber hot-water bottle on top of a ticking alarm clock, and he sleeps like the dead.

Dog's Dinner

OUR new budgerigar arrived the other day and has ingratiated himself with the entire family—except for our cocker spaniel, who spends all his waking hours with his eyes fixed unblinkingly on the newcomer, attempting to teleport it out of the cage and into his throat.

This is not surprising in view of his general attitude towards our feathered friends. The oyster-catchers on the river bank rise in noisy hysteria as he approaches at 40 mph, and though the rooks and black-headed gulls are less impressionable, having seen this sort of thing many times before, they too are panicked by the steam-engine panting, the thundering feet, and the slavering jaws. In the winter time he prowls round the bird tables in the neighbourhood, partly to eat the crumbs of bread underneath, but also in the hope that one of the patrons might have fallen off and sustained a quadriplegia.

He has reduced the rabbits in the wood to a state of terror—not that he ever catches one, for his technique precludes this. When a rabbit crosses his path he invariably follows the scent back to where the rabbit came from, not towards its destination. Such defeats are accepted philosophically, as the operation of a mysterious fate.

Dead rabbits are easier prey, but something of a nuisance, since when seized they have to be buried as near to the spot as practicable, and this may take a long time. Easier still are the remains of picnics; cast-off sandwiches can be disentangled from their wrappings, and on red-letter days there may even be a chocolate bar. Every now and then he finds a large soup bone, for there is a bone club among the local dogs. Bones are carried round the circuit and discarded when they become too heavy; they are then picked up by the next dog passing, and so on.

Similar finds are uncommon indoors, where food is kept out of reach and the penalties for stealing are severe. Yesterday morning, however, Homer nodded, and a whole family-size loaf left unguarded on the kitchen table was abstracted and consumed; the peristalsis which followed could be heard in the next room.

We attribute this episode to stress induced by the incursion of the budgie, and await with some anxiety the advent of a birthday hamster which is due in a few days' time.

Dog vs. Newspaper

WHEN I tidied up the garage recently I found a tin of flea powder we bought many years ago for the dog we had at that time. 'Stand Dog on Newspaper' began the instructions peremptorily, thereby betraying the fact that, however much R. & D. had gone into the product, no field work had ever been done.

In the first place Dog, though perhaps no genius in other aspects of daily life, can recognise a game when he sees one. Initially he is full of enthusiasm, trying to grab Newspaper, tear a large piece off, and run with it all over the garden. (Most of Dog's repertoire of games involve running, very seldom in the direction of other players.) It takes two, or perhaps three, people to convince Dog that no game is intended, and that this is all deadly earnest. Once this penetrates, nothing will induce Dog to approach Newspaper; he has to be lugged protestingly into position, scuffling Newspaper into a crumpled mass.

After Newspaper has been spread out again, Dog gets the idea that his tormentors wish to scratch his stomach, and rolls over, half on and half off Newspaper, with his feet in the air. This exposes his Eyes to potential contact with Powder, which is Dangerous. Exhortation and threats alike fail to stimulate Dog to change position, and it becomes necessary to turn him upright by main force, two people holding the bows and two the stern, while the fifth attempts to sprinkle on Powder. By this time Newspaper has been reduced to lacework, and the first touch of Powder on Dog's back confirms his impression that personal space is being violated; the resultant convulsions totally demolish what is left of Newspaper. Most of Powder is distributed over the five operators, who sneeze for hours, while Dog escapes between their feet to safety behind the shrubbery, where he evades capture indefinitely.

Our current Dog is prone to ticks, which can easily be dealt with by Spencer-Wells forceps or simply allowed to drop off on to the kitchen linoleum, where they are despatched by Dog himself; he has not yet been afflicted by fleas. However, I have kept the tin of flea powder; it is comforting to know that a thoroughly reliable remedy is at hand in case of emergency.

Bringing Up Butter

To the district council my dog is a creature loaded with *Toxocara*, helminths, and assorted pathogenic micro-organisms, ready, at the drop of a motion, to send senior citizens skidding into the orthopaedic ward and to blind every child within a radius of five miles. To express their disesteem and anxiety they have put up ubiquitous notices prohibiting the exercise of his excretory function, and to avoid severe financial penalities I am obliged to limit his daily walks to a disused railway line which serves as a social centre for the local dogs. To the west, where lie the snooty suburbs, the dogs look like type specimens of their breeds for the judges at Crufts, but if we turn east, towards the city, those we meet tend to look as though they had been assembled by photofit. I am glad to report that east or west is all the same to my dog, who competes in affability and excretion with the best, whether high or low.

I do not share the council's apprehension about the lower end of his alimentary canal, but the upper end is a different matter. There is, for example, a tendency towards hyperemesis after a surfeit of grass or other toxic material ingested during his walks. If this takes place on the kitchen floor it can be dealt with easily, but some time ago he stole a quarter of a pound of butter and produced it again on the living-room carpet—naturally, in a place where nobody could miss it. The problem of neutralising a butter induced lesion of this kind has proved baffling to a succession of domestic and professional experts, and my own repeated efforts, though apparently successful in the short term, have but a poor prognosis. Like Rizzio's blood in Holyrood, the mark returns, dark and shiny, and with a sinister and irregular outline, with every change in the weather or when guests are expected.

The other afternoon the health visitor, on her routine round of the wrinklies under her jurisdiction, dropped in to ask about my toenails. Her attention was not wholly on the matter in hand, for her gaze was fixed, not on my slippers, but, with ill-concealed distaste, on the stain. Somewhat abstractedly she made a number of notes on her pad, and I fear that among them must have been 'visit from social worker required'. I am buying a mat to cover my shame tomorrow.

The Trial

OUR glen is pretty isolated, and the inhabitants well scattered; the only rallying ground is the hotel, and apart from the weekly rounds of the fish van and the grocer there is little entertainment on offer. Accordingly the annual sheep-dog trials are a popular, though suitably serious, diversion. Entries are accepted from the two neighbouring glens as well as our own, and the function boasts a printed Order of Ballot, three cups, some money prizes, and an adjudicator imported from a respectable distance, so as to dispel any suspicion of favouritism.

This year, instead of the howling wind and horizontal sleet which outdoor activity normally attracts, there was lovely sunshine, and a large crowd of locals and visitors came to watch. City slickers wishing to place bets must have been mildly confused by the fact that 4 of the 18 dogs were called Don and 3 were named Spot, while 3 of the shepherds were Macdonalds and 2 were Turnbulls. The locals could, of course, name the entire ancestry and the current relatives of both dogs and men, as well as predict their likely performance.

The task was the standard one, points being awarded for outrun, lift, fetch, drive, pen, and shed, and at first all went smoothly. Successive batches of forlorn and bemused sheep were fetched, driven through gates, and round the specified course, finally being penned to public acclamation. But with the third Don, routine was disrupted. His master came to the starting post, indicated the 3 sheep standing disconsolately in the distance, and gave the dog the necessary command. Immediately the animal, clearly in rude health, willing and eager to give of his best, ran and ran and ran, totally ignoring the sheep, and vanished over the hill towards the sunset. The shepherd, after several vain and blasphemous attempts to recall him, finally turned to the judge and said, more in sorrow than in anger, 'That'll be it, then, Jim.'

The incident reminded me forcefully of the innumerable times I have urged my students to *read the question* before wildly starting to write, usually without any regard to what the examiner had in mind.

Animal Fancier

A friend of ours recently returned from a somewhat trying social weekend spent at a house where they keep a herd of yellow cats for decorative purposes. The doyen of the establishment, a large and cynical tom, had of late taken to looking on the place merely as a sort of second-rate hotel serving indifferent meals. He now lived in the rafters of a disused outhouse, and visited the house at rare intervals, speaking to no-one. It was generally felt that the animal was not pulling its weight, and our friend, stamped as an animal fancier because of his knowledge of the internal economy of the Wistar rat, was deputed to catch the cat to take him to the vet to be destroyed. Physiologists are brave enough in a reckless sort of way, and our friend accepted the commission. Armed only with a cardboard hatbox and his personality, he approached his quarry during its siesta by means of a long ladder. The cat observed the operation dreamily, and such was the lethargy induced by its excesses of the previous night that, after a purely formal protest which caused our friend to fall headlong down four rungs and nearly lost him the sight of one eye, it suffered itself to be placed in the hatbox, secured with string, and settled on the back seat of the car.

By the first traffic lights it had become clear that the cat, though tolerant of hatboxes, thought nothing of cars, and was taking itself to task for allowing itself to be imposed upon. At the second traffic lights our friend looked round in response to a sinister tearing noise and observed a yellow eye regarding him balefully through a jagged hole in the hatbox. Before any steps could be taken, the animal had become fully abreast of the situation and emerged as if propelled by a blasting charge. Our friend tells us that the car became full of cats, thereby causing him to reconsider his views on mammalian parthenogenesis in hatboxes; he counted at least fifteen as they flashed past, upsetting ashtrays, disrupting upholstery, and dismantling armrests. Finally one of the multitude landed squarely on the top of our friend's head and shot out of the driving window, leaving the car empty. By the time he had staunched his shredded scalp and returned home the cat was once more in residence in the outhouse and taking a well-earned nap.

The atmosphere at supper was rather chilly, and our friend's reputation as an animal fancier is now confined to the Wistar rat.

Cat Burglar

A recent Parliamentary answer reported in the papers has assured me that in Britain between 1981 and 1985 only one person was killed by a cat. But though the mortality from this cause appears to be low, no mention was made of the morbidity, which may well be more significant.

My daughter was recently given an Abyssinian kitten, a beautiful and most affectionate animal, with a disconcerting habit of sitting bolt upright and looking exactly like an ancient Egyptian god. Apart from an initial doubt whether it should properly be addressed in Amharic, good relations were at once established and the kitten was much admired. However, it turned out that no fewer than three of my daughter's friends were unable to visit the house without being overtaken by an acute allergic rhinitis, so that her party-giving activities were considerably impeded.

This problem did not affect me when I went to stay, and the kitten transferred some of its amiability to me, purring thunderously on my lap and rubbing its head energetically against any available portion of my anatomy. But matters did not stop there, and there were sudden springs on my back during meals and unexpected blast-offs from my thighs at other times. In every case the needle sharp claws tore shorts, trousers, and flesh impartially, and since I was on warfarin at the time the theoretical possibility of cat scratch fever was compounded by considerable messy effusion of blood.

Worse was to come. I have a small dental plate bearing three front teeth, of little functional but considerable decorative value, and several times during my visit I observed the kitten on the bedside table patting these teeth in a meditative way with its paws. On my last morning there I emerged from the shower to find that the kitten had made off with my teeth and hidden them so securely that three intensive searches of the house and garden failed to discover any trace of them.

That, of course, was the morning the photographer came to immortalise me for the benefit of the department in which I used to work. The session went ahead, but I am told that none of the pictures was satisfactory. After a month my teeth have still not surfaced, and I have had to get some more.

My dentist thinks all this is rather comical (as well as profitable), more particularly since my previous plate was chewed and eaten by my puppy.

Hippophobia

A friend of ours who dabbles in psychiatry recently purchased a young horse, partly in order that his waist-line could be held to the limits of his present wardrobe, and partly so that his children could add equitation to their other numerous accomplishments. The animal has taken charge of the household very satisfactorily, and apart from a tendency to request admission to the warmth of the kitchen fire at inopportune moments, has settled in well. For some time now our friend has been superintending the erection of a covered shelter of concrete blocks to protect the horse from the inclemencies of the English winter, and in this charitable work he has been assisted by a youth who has an aptitude for the compounding of concrete but little talent for conversation. On several occasions our friend has observed the youth and the horse eyeing each other with undisguised apprehension, and finally he taxed his helper with an un-English lack of sympathy with the great family of *Equidae*. The unnatural boy readily agreed. 'You see,' he explained, 'my mother was frightened by a horse before I was born.'

The Pacer

A preclinical friend of ours spent much of his boyhood on a farm, and later lived for some years next door to a riding stable. In spite of these formative influences he often used to assure us that he could take horses or leave them alone. Indeed, when he heard that his daughter had become the owner of half a standard horse, his pulse did not quicken nor did his pupils dilate. His only immediate reaction was to wonder whether it was the front or the back half of the animal that had joined the family. However, on reflection he decided that it would be only civil to pay a call on his daughter's acquisition when next he visited her.

It would be hard to say at what point his attitude of indifference changed. Perhaps it was when the horse, on being introduced, presented its rump to him to be scratched. Perhaps it was later, at the first harness race meeting he had ever attended. He found himself immersed in an ambience of bell boots and knee boots, head checks and huples, and though the commentator's use of phrases like 'taking the breeze', 'boiling over', or 'keeping him honest' conveyed but little, he did learn something about the American sulky and the Australian spider, and how to discard both terms in favour of the in-word 'cart'. He was apprised of the value of shorteners, and acquired a second-hand contempt for 'mere galloping races' as opposed to the mystique of pacing.

Now that he is back at work our friend often visualises the gallant animal pounding along towards victory, and, with a lamentable lack of insight, regards it as a potential saviour of the family finances. Unfortunately for this theory the horse's IQ is well down among the lower centiles, and the raising of the starting gate usually leaves it looking wildly round while the opposition disappears into the middle distance. This basic defect has so far not been remedied, and in addition the horse, when not in spreaders, is prone to kick itself savagely, so becoming incapacitated for months at a time. Its true value to our friend is therefore not as a winner of races, but as a topic of conversation at morning tea; his more innocent subordinates now consider him to be a sound judge of horseflesh. Last week his junior research assistant invited him to help with the local gymkhana.

Discourse with a Sheep

ON holiday this year a friend of ours found that at the farm where he frequently stays there had been an addition to the nominal roll of the household. The newcomer was a half-grown sheep, blind from birth, which had been rescued as a lamb by the young son of the house. The animal's allotted task was to keep down the grass in the garden, and it spent its nights in the garden shed. While in the shed it maintained a discreet silence, but while working it delivered an unending series of plaintive and piercing bleats; it was impossible to hold a conversation with anyone within ten yards of the epicentre. Fortunately the sheep could be temporarily turned off by the voice of its rescuer, and a tape recording of his voice making soothing noises and encouraging remarks had been rigged up on a long lead into the garden, where it was played whenever it was desirable for human discussions to take place.

Our friend had lunch with the family on the garden table, with a small dog and a cat, both old retainers, sleeping alongside him, the tape recorder in action, and the sheep nuzzling quietly round underneath, looking for its benefactor.

In spite of this relief, the penetrating vocalisation which punctuated the rest of the day whenever the tape recorder was switched off took toll of our friend's nerves, which were considerably jangled when he retired to bed.

Whether because of the sheep or for other reasons the cat, like our friend, spent a disturbed night. Not only did it stamp around in the passage like its counterpart in P.G. Wodehouse, but at 0430 h it transferred its activity to the keys of the piano, producing a loud and unearthly sonatina suggestive of the influence of Pierre Boulez, and banishing any further thought of sleep.

We understand from our friend that he is thinking of giving the farm a miss until the sheep has become mutton and the musical aspirations of the cat have been sublimated in some other direction.

John and Mery

IT is now some weeks since our hamsters were installed. They live in a glass-fronted case in one of the bedrooms, where they may be seen, dim shapes behind the murky glass. Their presence, however, permeates the house, and they are consulted on all domestic affairs and also on matters of more general interest, such as the probability of snow on Christmas Day.

Even more immanent than their own corporeal existence are the countless generations of unborn hamsters due to spring from their loins, and so many of these have been given away already that the market is saturated. Their slightest gesture is interpreted as a sign of incipient maternity, as, for example, when one of them bit a too-familiar visitor to the effusion of blood, and the action was held to show its highly nervous state; or when the other was observed to demolish three cheese biscuits in rapid succession and its perverted appetite was assumed to demonstrate its delicate condition.

Though surrounded by every luxury, they are determined to escape, and spend the watches of the night in scratching holes in odd corners. They have already spent one night at large, and we await with some trepidation their next eruption. A large notice has in fact been erected on the cage which reads 'Hamsters, John and Mery, Pleese be ceful.'

Language Lessons

ALL this chat that is going on about the identification of human intersexes by skin biopsy and examination of the polymorphs prompts us to publicise the case of our budgerigar. Two years ago the thought came to us that the long winter evenings of our declining years might be enlivened if we had a budgerigar to recite to us. When we get tired of Pop Goes the Weasel, we thought, we will switch him on to Mary had a Little Lamb, and when the sentiments of Rockabye Baby have begun to cloy we will teach him Pat-a-cake, Pat-a-cake, Baker's Man. Right, then, we said, we shall buy a budgerigar.

When we brought him home he was surrounded by quantities of budgerigar seed, a supply of golden budgerigar sand, a small sack of budgerigar grit, and a packet of budgerigar cuttlefish bone (packed on the sun-drenched uplands and full of budgerigar vitamins). Also we had a small budgerigar booklet. 'Male birds,' said the budgerigar booklet on p. 1, 'can be identified by the blue colour of the mask at the base of the beak (see illust., Fig. 1).' We looked at Billy (he had been christened in the car). Sure enough his mask was a pale blue and entirely consonant with the appearances as shown in illust., Fig. 1. Having satisfied ourselves that the new member of the household was indeed a male, and therefore a born entertainer, we expended some thousands of invaluable man-hours, to say nothing of woman-hours and child-hours, in trying to get his name through our budgerigar's ivory skull. 'Billy!' we would begin patiently over the breakfast table in a level calm voice designed to inspire confidence. 'Billy!!' we cried jocularly over lunch: 'Billy!' we croaked hoarsely at supper. 'Billy!!!' we roared at bedtime when our control had begun to crack.

After six months of nervous and laryngeal exhaustion, during which our budgerigar consumed several pounds of budgerigar seed, a mountain of budgerigar grit, and a small fortune in sun-drenched cuttlefish bones, we observed that his mask was changing colour to medium brown. A horrible suspicion seized us, and we dived at once into our budgerigar booklet. Yes, our suspicions were well founded. Billy's mask no longer corresponded to illust., Fig. 1, but was in all respects identical with illust., Fig. 2. The matter was clinched the other day when he won second prize as a female in the miscellaneous Class of our local R.S.P.C.A. show. (First was a guineapig we know well, from down the road).

Our concept of our budgerigar as an accomplished diseur (or even diseuse) has been abandoned, and we are reconciled to spending our declining years in the company of a series of deafening feminine steam-whistle cheeps. But we must confess we find the whole thing rather disturbing. We think perhaps it must have been that nasty thermonuclear stuff that did it.

Saturnalia in a Garage

A friend of ours is the proud owner of two delicately nurtured female cats of tender years, and he has been at pains to prevent their characters becoming warped by a premature acquaintance with the opposite sex. The other evening, observing an expectant circle of tom cats in the back yard, he formed the opinion that his protective care was needed, and craftily took evasive action by shutting up his innocent charges in the garage.

In the morning he visited the garage before breakfast, to reassure its occupants. As he opened the door two bedraggled, bleary-eyed objects crept unsteadily out, followed at a stately pace by a large black tom, licking his chops, who had been carefully locked in with them by mistake.

The Holocaust

A clinical friend of ours has for some time been dabbling in Science on a part-time basis – three afternoons a month, we think it is. He has often told us that the experience is proving mildly discouraging. He potters about the lab., and every now and then he writes down some results, but it never seems to come to anything. When he embodies his findings in a paper it excites nationwide apathy. If only he could have a Break-through, he says, like all these F.R.S. chaps.

When we met our friend the other day we saw at once that something had happened, and we pressed him to tell us about it. It appears that his kitchen had recently become invaded by ants. His normal reaction to ants is a rather colourless one, and he was not originally committed to an emotional viewpoint. At the urgent behest of his wife he absently sprayed the premises at intervals with insecticide, without observing any sensible diminution in the marching and counter-marching on the floor. One evening, however, as our friend was negligently toying with a slice of cherry cake, his teeth met in a small cluster of ants, torpid with strawberry jam. At one stroke his sensibilities became engaged, and he threw all the resources of a part-time scientist into the battle with a will. He devised traps; he stood the furniture in water; he built ramparts of strange proprietary powders. After he had wrought in this fashion for several days the volume of ants had increased slightly and the biscuit tin had fallen to the invaders. The honour of Science was at stake. Now mark what follows very closely.

It seems that on the shelf of our friend's kitchen there stands a round cardboard box which originally contained sulphadiazine. For some time, however, this box has been the repository of an indeterminate number of Tabs. Ventolin 2 mg, with which our friend is wont to solace his asthmatic dependants. Last year, when his anxiety neurosis was bad, our friend popped in some Tabs. diazepam 5 mg, and recently his wife took to keeping her paracetamol in the same place. There are also some oval pink things of whose nature our friend is uncertain, and a partly decomposed amorphous mass which he identifies as of antihista-minic origin.

Last week his wife was away from home, and our friend had to cook his breakfasts. One morning as he waited for the frying-pan to come to the sizzle, he picked up the box in the hope of finding a jujube which might temporarily stay his hunger. Judge of his emotion when he found the box filled with a pile of small black carcasses, every one stone dead.

Our friend is calmly confident; it only remains to identify the pink things and the rest will follow. He tells us that he has already enquired about the procedure at the Nobel prizegiving, and he loftily awaits the obsequious approach of B.B.C. 2.

Plagues

AN academic friend of ours who emigrated to Australia some time ago was recently on study leave, and was at pains to inform us that he had never worried about white ants. He had been on a trip up North, and had noted the acreage of scrub devoted to the North/South oriented termite mounds, but had not connected their inhabitants with his own civilized and leafy garden in the middle of the city. His happy state of mind was abruptly shattered when one morning he put his finger through the surround of the lavatory door, disclosing a mass of tunnels and an immense activity. Being ignorant of the proper procedure, he did not pretend he had not noticed and send for the pest control officer, who could have inserted poison bait for them to take to the queen. Instead, he indignantly tore off a large piece of wood, leaving the ants in no doubt they were discovered and stimulating them to scarper.

The expert he called in could not find the source anywhere in our friend's garden or those of his neighbours, but undertook to provide prophylaxis against further depredations.

Subsequently a confident but serious minded man ripped out all the infested wood and cut great holes in the floor, under which he crawled around on his stomach with a long spray attachment and an electric lantern. When he came to a difficult bit he sought comfort in singing evangelical hymns at the top of his voice. It was hard to concentrate on examination papers while 'Throw out the lifeline, someone is sinking today!' reverberated through the floorboards.

Eventually our friend's family was pronounced fit to live in their house again, free from fear, and immediately they were invaded by large numbers of mice which would pop their heads out of the oven, or climb cheekily on the draining board during washing up. These were followed in turn by a community of small frogs with voices like factory hooters, which surrounded the house to serenade the occupants during the hours of darkness.

Our friend has no cattle which could suffer from a murrain, and so far his family is clear of lice, boils and pestilence, but there have been thunderstorms with showers of enormous hailstones, and he is sure the flies are just as bad as they can have been in biblical Egypt. He confidently expects a plague of locusts at any moment, and is taking special care of his first-born.

In Transit

Happy Traveller

UNLIKE some people who are described as indefatigable travellers, I am eminently defatigable, and long-distance air travel in economy class is a weird I dislike having to dree. My flights always seem to start late at night, and however soon I check in all the decent seats have already gone. It is my routine fate to be sandwiched between a chap with the build of an all-in wrestler and a bulging female of some 95 kg; my thighs, which are 10 cm longer than the distance to the seat in front, become painfully wedged against the inflight literature. A couple of seats away will be a baby which cries intermittently all night, and in the row behind is a couple with a reversal of the sleep rhythm conversing in loud hoarse voices. The bladder problems of the all-in wrestler necessitate periodic upheavals, and small children race up and down the aisle screaming for free Coca-Cola.

The alcohol trolleys hold up the incessant traffic of exercise-minded passengers, and those so obstructed seek stability by lurching over to grab the back of my seat, causing a minor backlash injury. The issue of headsets is followed by an unwanted second dinner at 0200 h local time, and thereafter the first movie (which I cannot see, my seat being in the same plane as the screen) is succeeded by the duty-free shopping half-hour. It is true that after this there is a remote chance of briefly knitting up my ravelled sleeve of care, but the onset of stage-4 sleep is usually rent by the voice of the Captain, calm and reassuring, warning of approaching turbulence. Only too often he is right, and all hope of repose is finally knocked on the head by the issue of orange juice, followed by breakfast.

The daylight hours which follow are the reverse of remedial. A refuelling stop means further commotion and exhortation, a mass exodus and re-entry, energetic vacuum-cleaning, and noisy replacement of supplies of food and drink. My female neighbour inevitably requires help, in a foreign language, with the completion of her landing card, and when, after some 20 hours, I totter out, profoundly jet-lagged, it is to find that my suitcase is in the very last batch to be unloaded, and that the queue I have joined for immigration is hopelessly blocked by a couple attempting to enter the country illegally.

As a student I used to complain about being up all night with a midwifery case, but those were happy days, before I had any experience of life at 33000 feet.

Opinion Poll

WE have a medical friend who has several times credibly informed us that he had never had his opinion publicly polled, and when we met him the other day he was at pains to tell us that this stigma had now been removed. The great moment arrived as he was sitting peaceably in the Union Station in mile-high Denver, waiting for the Rocky Mountain Rocket to bear him away to Chicago. He tells us he was approached by a young lady bearing a bulging despatch case, who sat down beside him. 'I'm not trying to sell anything.' said the young lady hastily, with a trace of discomposure, 'I'm a public-opinion poll, and would you care to answer some questions?' Our friend was at once in the picture, and leaned forward eagerly, his tongue trembling with the urgency of his opinions on mile-high Denver, the British National Health Service, and the decadence of the Broadway theatre.

The young lady opened her bag and with difficulty extricated a large pile of dilapidated trade periodicals with titles like *Aluminum* and the *Precision Blockmaker's Weekly*. 'There,' she said, 'have you read any of these in the last week?' Our friend admitted his oversight, but excused it by his foreign origin. 'My!' exclaimed the young lady, 'to think I'm listening to the tongue Shakespeare spoke! It always gives me a kinda cold feeling right here!' She indicated the back of a shapely neck, and gazed in admiration at our friend, who had not appreciated his linguistic capabilities in this light before. It was with difficulty that the young lady remembered the rest of her mission, and produced for our friend's inspection a number of packs of cigarettes of all degrees of magnitude from Bantam to King-size. Our friend was forced to admit that as a non-smoker he could offer no constructive opinion on them, and the poll was over, leaving behind it on both sides a sense of mild frustration.

Determined that the young lady should have his opinion on some subject, our friend hazarded his belief that taking public-opinion polls in the Union Station in mile-high Denver must be an arduous occupation. His interlocutor agreed. 'But you should see me next week,' she said, 'I'm doing girdles and bras'.

To his lasting regret, our friend couldn't make it.

Travel Sickness

A peripatetic physician we know is a connoisseur of travel sickness, and is himself a distinguished executant. In his time he has utilised the receptacles provided by British, American, Swiss, and Australian civil airlines, and the floors provided by American and Australian military aircraft. On land his record is hardly less impressive: he has christened the interiors of numerous ambulances as far apart as Dublin and Salt Lake City, and in the bad old days before he became a joint owner of the concern, he made his mark one stormy night in the corridor of an L.M.S. express between Carlisle and Lockerbie. At sea he claims the Indian Ocean, the Great Australian Bight, the North Sea, and the Channel as certainties, and the Irish Sea and Mediterranean as probables (there was a high wind blowing at the time). Curiously enough, however, he had never been sick in the Atlantic, and the other day he took ship to rectify the omission.

For the first three hours his ambition was thwarted by the unreasonable placidity of the water, but at last the great moment arrived, and our friend strode proudly to the rail. His chagrin may be imagined when he found that the ocean was reserved for first-class passengers and that he was separated from it on all sides by no-man's-land containing life-boats. The train of events set in motion proved irreversible, and ultimately involved the ignominious use of one of the square buckets thoughtfully provided by the management in the more mobile parts of the vessel.

Our friend spent the rest of the trip in his bunk, surly and frustrated, rousing himself intermittently for his hyoscine. But he is not so easily beaten. He writes us from New York that he intends to charter a speedboat at Miami.

Passage of Time

IT is probably true that the activities of Mr. William Willett have been on balance beneficial to the country, but in at least one household they have left a legacy of confusion and despair. We can never find the paragraph in the papers which tells us whether to put the clocks forward or back, and if we once falter in our empirical belief and sit down to argue the matter out we are irretrievably lost. In fact, we have to get up unreasonably early on Sunday morning to find out from the B.B.C. whether or not we are two hours wrong.

All this is, of course, child's play to the Americans. We recently attempted a journey by rail from Cincinnati to Chicago, where we were to catch a plane. We were fresh and fit when we reached the travel agency, and we had a little notebook to take it all down in. It was not till we were immersed in schedules that we realised we were travelling on the day summer-time reached Chicago, but not Cincinnati. The young lady was most helpful. We would leave Cincinnati on Eastern Standard Time, but at Chicago we would be on Central Standard Time, so that normally we would have to put our watch back an hour. 'But then,' she said, 'Chicago will be on summer-time, so you'll have to put it right on again.' We were immediately roused. 'Well, then,' we said, 'what time is the time we are due to arrive in Chicago written in?' 'Central Standard, I guess,' said the young lady doubtfully, 'I don't know much about trains myself.' She rummaged in the back of the schedule. 'Yes,' she said, 'Central Standard.' 'So,' we said craftily, 'the train journey will actually take an hour longer than we think it will—or will it?' The young lady smiled patiently. 'You won't have to alter your watch will you?' she said, speaking slowly and distinctly. 'No,' we replied thankfully. 'Well, then,' she said, 'it will be an hour later than that time on your watch.' 'We see,' we said slowly (we really thought we did). 'Then how long will we have in Chicago till the plane leaves?' 'Ah,' said the young lady in a businesslike fashion, 'planes are different. We'll have to see what time your airline is operating on. Where did you say you were going?' We told her, and she had begun to look it up when a thought struck her, 'They'll be on Mountain Time, you know,' she said, 'and that means you'll have to put your watches back two hours instead of one before you get there. Unless, or course, they're having summer-time too . . .'

We staggered out, our spirit broken. When the time came, we turned up an hour too soon at Cincinnati.

Carrying Angles

ERGONOMICS does not seem to me to have progressed very far when it comes to suitcases. When I stand upright with my arm by the side and relaxed, the front end of a stick carried loosely in my hand points inwards at 45° and downwards and forwards at about 30°; this is the position of rest. Holding the stick horizontal and pointing directly forwards for any length of time imposes a slight but noticeable strain on the muscles and ligaments of virtually the whole upper limb. Yet this is how I have to carry heavy suitcases, sometimes for long periods, and much fatigue might be avoided if their handles were angled inwards and tilted downwards. However, symmetry would then require left-handed and right-handed suitcases.

This objection would disappear if the handle were made reversible. I cannot think of a way to construct a satisfactory stable tilting handle which would be easily and quickly reversible, but it would surely be possible to meet the need for reversibility in the horizontal plane. One solution would be to attach the handle, not directly to the suitcase, but to a flat rectangular metal bar 1–1.5 cm wide pivoted on the case at its centre. This bar would rotate under two flat semicircular metal 'bridges' firmly attached to the suitcase fore and aft of the pivot and centred on it. The bearing surfaces of the bar and the bridges could be slightly corrugated to prevent inadvertent slippage when taking the weight. The length of bridge necessary to allow the bar a range of 90° naturally depends on the diameter of the imaginary circle of which they are a part; if this is too great the length becomes inconveniently big, and if too short the stability of the arrangement is imperilled. With a compromise diameter of 8 cm the chord between the ends of each bridge would be about 6 cm.

Shopping baskets and pails present further problems, but certainly the flexible plastic handles which bunch the fingers painfully should be banned. Rectangular shopping baskets with rigid sides, or at least with rigid supporting bars bounding the aditus, could be fitted with two D-rings on each long side. This would allow a detachable handle to be fitted diagonally at 45°, and if the handle were equipped with spring clips like those on a dog lead it could be reversed with little trouble.

I should like to see a pail with a flattened side or sides to enable it to be carried with the arm vertical instead of painfully abducted; a similar arrangement of D-rings could than apply. However, such shapes are said to produce turbulence in the contents of the pail.

I have put these points to a series of highly qualified scientists and engineers, and have to report a virtual explosion of apathy. But I still think that there must be a better way to carry things. Perhaps readers could apply their minds to the problem?

Hunt the Indian

RECENTLY we heard from a chap we know who has made the medical grand tour of the United States. He is a family man, and it seems he embarked with strict instructions from his small son to establish contact at all costs with a Red Indian. The assignment, which seemed to present no difficulties at the Ocean Terminal at Southampton, proved a tough proposition. The medical schools he visited were situated in uncompromisingly Caucasian surroundings, and he was unable to locate a single tepee. At one Western school he inquired of his host how his mission could be accomplished. 'You'd better come down to the clinic tomorrow,' he said, 'the head nurse is an Indian'. Our friend explained that this was scarcely what he had in mind, and that his requirements included social as well as ethnological factors. The specifications imposed on him had been rather stringent, and only a Heap Big Chief with a hint of tomahawks and scalps in the background would suffice. The sort of man, in fact, who could only be properly addressed as 'How!' His mentor shook his head sadly. 'You're too early,' he said, 'they're not out yet. Tell you what, though,' he added, brightening, 'I can do you some Mexican Indians.' After some discussion it was felt that this would be cheating, and our friend, a man of some moral rectitude, was forced to decline. At Denver, however, he was able to arrange a trip to Buffalo Bill's grave, where he expended some wampum on photographic evidence of his good intentions.

In his subsequent visits our friend found himself staying at hotels within the jurisdiction of Crees, Iroquois, Blackfeet, and Senecas, but his sleep was undisturbed by a single war-whoop, and no solitary smoke signal caught his eye. His personality is of the ulcer-forming type, and his obligations began to prey on his mind. He became pale and worn, and even an encounter with a drugstore Indian in Baltimore did little to restore his spirits. Finally he had to embark with his mission unaccomplished, and at his reunion with his family he could not look his son in the eye. 'By the way,' he said later, 'I never saw that Indian of yours.' 'Didn't you?' said his taskmaster indifferently. 'Daddy, how many propellers has the *Queen Mary*?'

Chlorophyll

DURING the chlorophyll promotion of the fifties a medical friend of ours who was visiting the United States had the misfortune to run out of toothpaste in Iowa. At the nearest drug-store he shouldered his way past the Kwik Lunch counter, the toys, the telephones, and the Bantam Books, and found himself in the dim atmosphere of that submerged appendix to the establishment, the counter marked Chemicals, Biologicals, Cut-Rate Drugs. 'Why, hello there!' said the young lady behind the counter, delighted to assist our friend's deliberations. He intimated his desires, and the young lady indicated a vast pile of assorted toothpaste, all as green as grass. Our friend's Scottish blood rose to take command. 'Yes,' he said, 'but do you have any without chlorophyll?' A visible shudder ran through the young lady, and her manner became cold and distant. 'I guess so,' she said doubtfully, and disappeared into the back of the store. She was absent for several minutes, giving our friend time to contemplate a notice reading 'America's *Finest* Vitamin.' Eventually she returned, bearing a dusty and rather battered package, which she handled with evident distaste; it was clear she was going to apply for danger money that very afternoon. However, the contents were indeed toothpaste, and after scrutinising the tube to make sure it incorporated no Cut-Rate Drugs or Biologicals our friend handed over the money in a chilly silence and withdrew.

It was only after he got around to cleaning his teeth with the stuff that he found it was flavoured with beechnut—a taste he particularly dislikes—and that in the stress of the moment he had bought, not a King-size, not a Giant-size, but a Zombie-size tube, enough to last him for several years.

Sanitary Resting

'BUT what about the plumbing?' we asked the returned traveller impatiently; 'tell us about the plumbing.' Our friend obligingly rehearsed to us his encounters with dish-washing machines and garbage-disposal units: his eyes bulged dutifully, but it was plain his thoughts were elsewhere. He came round to it in the end. It was in Cleveland, he said, that his host took him for half an hour to visit a bowling alley. After watching the automatic re-setting machine (our friend is in some respects a simple man) in a happy daze for some ten minutes, his eye fell on a notice in the corner saying 'Sanitary Rest Rooms,' and, feeling in need of a sanitary rest, he took himself off. He had, he said, expected the Usual Offices, and it is important that this attitude be borne in mind in view of what followed. The room, he said, was full of a vicious blue light emanating from behind the throne. He took hold of the seat and pulled it forward; there was a click and the light disappeared, only to return with a splutter when he released his hold and the power-driven seat rose slowly and majestically on its well-oiled bearings to its former vertical position. Our friend is not an electronics man, but he spent an exciting few minutes exploring the machine for evidences of negative feed-back before he discovered a little notice reading 'This seat is sterilized in 60 seconds.' In short, he had found a Sewage Disposal Unit.

This, then, was the high spot of his trip. It is true that subsequently he patronised Clean Sanitary Rest Rooms, Rest Rooms with Sanitary Seat Covers, and on one occasion even a Hygienic Sanitary Rest Room. In Chicago he found the seat encircled by a paper tape of the kind used to open bridges, bearing red crosses and the motif 'Sterilised for *Your* Protection' worked tastefully in green, and in New York he explored the gigantic underground establishment in Radio City Music Hall with television laid on. He even visited Hygiene, Colo. But it is to Cleveland that his admiration goes; he tells us he is thinking of starting a bowling alley underneath our museum.

Ticks

THE other day we ventured to envy a colleague of ours his recent trip to America. He would have none of it. 'Nothing but devilish hard work', he said, flushing under his copper-coloured sun-tan, 'no time to enjoy myself at all.' We stood him a drink, and his attitude modified slightly. He had, it appeared, just snatched a few moments to see Niagara Falls, and had allowed himself to be persuaded into a baseball game or two for a couple of seconds. He had seen the Kentucky Derby and George Washington's bowling green, and, protesting vigorously the while, had suffered himself to be transported across Lake Champlain in a ferry boat. Finally, he had been taken up the Rocky Mountains in the car of an amiable bacteriologist who is also a mountaineer.

At the outset the bacteriologist clicked his tongue over our friend's city slicker shoes: 'We can't do much for you in these', he said sadly. As the car climbed the foothills another thought struck him. 'By the way', he said, 'You'd better tuck your trousers into you socks when we get off the trail. This is the bad season for them.' 'Bad season?' queried our friend. 'The ticks, you know', said the bacteriologist impatiently, wrenching the offside wheel back from the edge of a precipice. 'Of course', he said reassuringly, as he changed gear, 'we don't have anything like the mortality here they do up North. Some places it's over ninety per cent, but here we only run about fifty.' A chill little wind from the snowy peaks crept in through the car window and played on our friend's neck; the sunshine hesitated. 'Of course', he agreed hollowly. 'You'll see them all right once they get on you', said the bacteriologist, 'they're quite big.' 'And of course', he added cheerfully, 'they don't always bite, and if they *do* bite they're not always infected. You don't have to *worry* about them.' He glanced complacently at his own thick puttees.

'There's another thing too', said the bacteriologist informatively, 'you'll probably feel like death tomorrow. The altitude doesn't get you at the time, it's only later you feel it. Sometimes you get it at the time, though', he went on reminiscently, 'I remember the first time I climbed that fellow over there I was as sick as a dog on the top – nose and ears bleeding and so on.' He laughed happily at the memory. 'Today we're going to go right over the shoulder of it to that big one beyond. Incidentally, I remember having quite a nasty experience with a bear up there . . .'

Our friend tells us the thing he enjoyed most in America was the Empire State Building.

Life Upside Down

WHEN I was at school, I was much taken with the problem of how the Australians managed to conduct their affairs while suspended upside down. Sir maintained that they were really not upside down at all, but I was never convinced by this dogmatic statement (Sir had never been to Australia, so how did he know?)

Nowadays, when I visit Australia frequently, my original picture of Australian postural problems has been strongly reinforced. The sun, which in Scotland is wont to travel sedately from left to right as you look at it, in Australia rides round the course from right to left, causing untold alarm and despondency; at night the moon behaves in the same unnatural fashion. It is not seriously to be supposed that something has happened to the sun and moon, and only one explanation satisfies the facts; the Australians are upside down.

The shape of the moon confirms this. The Romans used to call it *luna mendax*, the lying moon, since when it was waxing (*crescens*) it was shaped like a 'D', and when it was waning (*decrescens*) it was shaped like a 'C'. Anything in the nature of a Latin mnemonic to describe its behaviour was thus impossible to formulate. But in Australia the waxing moon is C-shaped, and the waning moon is D-shaped, it is a truthteller, not a liar. These shapes can of course be reversed if the observer stands on his head, and the conclusion is once again inescapable; the Antipodes (for I generously include New Zealand) and their inhabitants must be upside down.

The meteorological implications of this inversion are interesting. It has long been received knowledge that the bath-water in the Northern hemisphere eddies out through the plug-hole in the reverse direction to that taken by the contents of Southern baths. But several eminent scientists of my acquaintance have made minute observations on their bath-water as they crossed the Equator, and have failed to detect any change. They have therefore concluded that in this one respect there is no distinction between Scotland and Australia. However, their opinion is founded on a faulty premise. What they have not realized is that after the Equator has been crossed the observer is upside down, and is therefore looking *up* to the plug-hole from below. Now a right to left swirl looked at from below is seen as a left to right swirl, and it follows that if the direction of the swirl in these experiments did not *appear* to change, this is excellent evidence that it *did* in fact change. There is thus a real difference between Northern and Southern baths.

Apart from these cosmic phenomena there are numerous petty mechanical difficulties associated with living upside down. For example, the grandfather clock I brought with me when I first settled in Australia obstinately refused to adapt itself to the altered gravitational field, and, in spite of being subjected to petrol baths and other indignities, maintained a sullen silence until I thought of the expedient of nailing one of its feet to the floor. Even then it sometimes struck thirteen about four o'clock in the morning.

Physiologically there is less to remark. For a few days after arrival in Australia I have a fuzzy feeling in my head which is qualitatively different from mere jet lag, such as I experience when travelling in the Northern hemisphere, and must be attributed to a readjustment of the circulation to prevent blood pooling in my brain. But I am soon able to cope with the incessant rush of blood to the head, and the difficulty of adjusting to the inverted image on the retina proves to be evanescent, though it sometimes returns temporarily after official dinner parties. But my sleep rhythm often becomes disturbed, for the roofs of Australian houses are the haunt of innumerable Australian cats, which nightly, like Macbeth, murder sleep. (Australian cats naturally gravitate to the roof rather than the floor, even though they have claws to hold them down).

All things considered, it is quite a relief to step on to the tarmac at Heathrow and find myself once again the right way up. But I do wish that the wretched place was less overcrowded and impersonal, and that it had a supply of Australian sunshine.

Cultural Exchange

WHEN we lived in Western Australia we used to get a bundle of British Sunday newspapers sent to us every few weeks. The time lag of six weeks or more took much of the urgency out of the news they contained, but we always enjoyed the magazine section; particularly the film reviews.

These were something of a lucky dip, since some of the films discussed did not arrive in Perth for at least a year after the review, by which time our memory of what it said was a little sketchy. But this delay could not be relied upon, and often we saw American films before London did, and British ones before New York. I am also tempted to say that we saw some Italian films which no-one else ever saw anywhere, even in Italy. These circumstances meant that we never knew whether we should find a critique of a picture we saw a couple of months ago, or one that was coming next week, or of one that never came at all. Nevertheless our enthusiasm was in no way diminished, for my wife and I were dedicated filmgoers.

Apart from the films, we got a great deal out of these Sunday papers – the news of books, the gramophone records, the local scandals and opinions – and were duly grateful. We often

wanted to make some sort of return for this flow of enlighten-
ment, but it was not until we had a letter from one of our friends
in Britain that we realized that we were already, and quite
unwittingly, making a substantial repayment.

At Christmas time we used to send our benefactors calendars
– the pictorial kind, with a different colour picture for each
month. The general scheme of such calendars is much the same
everywhere, but there was a particular magic in sending an
Australian one to Britain, for the seasons are reversed. A British
calendar in January is a cold thing to look at, for by some quirk
publishers think that people want to have on their walls the
same sort of weather they have outside the house. Accordingly,
during the long cold British winter they provide their customers
with pictures of snow and ice. The Australian pictures at this
time are very different – tropical bathing beaches, sunlit scrub,
flowering gums, and great herds of dusty cattle swimming
across tired-looking creeks. With this sort of thing to look at, our
friends felt, it would not be so long until Spring arrived to put
an end to the succession of dripping fogs and burst taps.

These calendars were just as important in the British summer,
so often dull, damp, cloudy and wholly disappointing. In all the
Australian pictures throughout the year the sun shines high in
the sky, the white light strikes downwards brilliantly, almost
hurting the eyes; it is impossible to look at this splash of
startling light, this warmth of vivid blue and red and brown,
without feeling cheered and hopeful.

This then, was what we unheedingly used to send to Britain
in return for our Sunday edification – we sent the sun into
people's houses, and they were happy in the exchange, for it is
a tremendous thing to have the sun in your house all the year
round.

Decline of Photography

WHEN I travel abroad I always take my camera with me, to
record scenery and events, with the everpresent possibility of
producing a masterpiece or two on the side. I used to take great
pleasure in doing this, scrambling about on the hillsides to get
the best angle and irritating my wife, who sat in the car tapping

her feet. But of late my satisfaction has become dimmed by the remorseless advance of electronic technology, which has taken most of the fun out of photography.

When I was eleven my mother (a fervent Presbyterian) won a box Brownie camera at a church raffle, and, being upset at acquiring something by this manifestly unChristian method, gave it to me, so that at least she personally would not benefit by her transgression.

I processed the films by see-sawing them in open dishes supported on tea-chests in a hermetically sealed store cupboard behind the kitchen. I rigged up a small torch bulb behind a red glass, but when panchromatic films came in I had to make do with total darkness. Initially I made prints on 'daylight' paper, setting up the printing frames at the windows of the sitting room. The gradual appearance of the brown image was a great thrill, and made it possible to judge the exposure exactly. But when I took to 'gaslight' paper it was more difficult; I had to light a measured length of magnesium ribbon in my store cupboard and hold it a fixed distance away from the paper. Much paper was spoiled by this procedure. Eventually the great day arrived when the house was wired for electricity, and life was transformed. I was given an enlarger, and won a prize in a competition.

When I was twenty I graduated to a second-hand early model Rolleiflex, and began to use various exposure and distance meters. Later, I experimented with the now defunct Dufay colour process in the dark-rooms of the University departments where I worked. It was the Rolleiflex (suitably taped up and sealed by the authorities to deceive the Japanese about my intentions) which accompanied me to tropical Queensland in the latter part of the war. In these days the production of acceptable negatives and prints from materials of doubtful stability in the heat and humidity of makeshift dark-rooms was an art in which the practitioner could take legitimate pride, and occasionally the hard-won results made me feel a kinship with the Victorian pioneers.

These intimations of immortality did not long outlast the war. I dropped the Rolleiflex, and it was never the same afterwards. The next step down the slippery slope was to buy a 35 mm camera with built-in exposure meter, and this in turn was superseded by another one equipped in addition with automatic wind and through the lens focusing. I now have no access to dark room facilities, and the only aspect of photography I can enjoy is composing the picture; everything else is done for me by arbitrarily imposed technology and impersonal commercial organizations. Perhaps I am out of step with progress, but I often look back to the kitchen cupboard very nostalgically.

The Diggings

WHEN my children were small they each possessed a small piece of quartz which at first sight appeared in no way distinguished. But protruding from each lump as though it had been fused on from outside, was a small irregularly shaped piece of gold, the size of a lentil. These nuggets, the pride of their lives, were given to them by a real live prospector in the great gold field which used to supply some eighty per cent of Australia's gold.

The trip from Perth to Kalgoorlie involves 372 miles of excellent bitumen road running first through the hills on to the great plateau, through the wheat belt, and finally into the low scrub which extends for hundreds of miles in all directions, broken only by rocky outcrops and salt pans which become lakes in the rainy season. Alongside the road, supported on concrete cradles, runs the goldfields water pipe from Mundaring Weir, twenty miles east of Perth. Sometimes the pipe gleams freshly silver, but for the greater part of its enormous length it is a dirty black and looks hot and tired. Beyond Southern Cross there are pumping stations at intervals along the track of the pipe – a couple of houses and a shed in the middle of nothing. The road shoots straight to the horizon, bordered by hard red gravel, and through the baked surface of this the wild flowers thrust up incredibly in yellows and blues and reds. You have five or ten miles notice of the approach of another car, so there is plenty of time to slow down from your lonely eighty or ninety miles an hour to a speed more suitable for company.

We took our time through the unfamiliar country, eating our meals by the side of the road and watching the price of petrol mount as we left the coast behind. Just beyond Coolgardie we stopped to cook our chops in the gathering dusk, quite unaware

that we were sitting on top of a gold mine, and had just begun
to spread ourselves and open our tin of cake when the miner
came stumping down from the little hill behind us, an elderly
man in navvy's trousers and a grey flannel shirt. We asked him
to sit and have a chop, and he sat down heavily, being stiff with
age and effort, and took some bread and cheese and tea. The
chop was too much for him, for he had no teeth, and after
watching him mumble it round in his mouth for some time we
suggested that he might like to take the left-overs and cook them
for himself the next day. He wrapped them up in an old piece
of newspaper and stuffed them in his pocket, and then showed
us where to find a little tap let into the enormous pipe on the
other side of the road; we had our first drink of goldfields water.

After supper he told us that he had been after gold for thirty
years. He had originally come from Shropshire, and had been
knocking about the goldfields ever since in one capacity or
another. He had signally failed to acquire an Australian accent,
and his soft voice sounded a little out of place in these harsh
surroundings. At the moment he was working all by himself,
and had struck a good patch. The mine had been through
several hands, and had more or less been given up, but he was
sure it had a lot of life in it yet. It was too dark for us to look
at it that night, but he asked us to come up and see it on our
way back from Kalgoorlie. We packed up our stuff and watched
him climb clumsily and slowly up the little hill as we left.

I had work to do in Kalgoorlie, but in the late afternoon of the
next day one of the local doctors had arranged for us to see over
the Lake View and Star, the biggest mine on the golden mile at
Boulder. Here was a very different aspect of gold mining – a
huge organization bringing up ore from nearly a mile below
the surface and processing it into gold. The massive power
house built of the ubiquitous corrugated iron contained enough
dynamos to supply a small city; the gigantic crushers and
roasting tanks occupied several acres; the winding machinery
was as impressive as any child could wish. The disappointment
was the stuff that came up from the depths – a dull grey rock
which arrived by the carload and was ground into an even
duller grey powder before being roasted into gold. Unfortunately it was not the day for pouring, which undoubtedly
would have stirred our imaginations, and so we carried away
with us an impression admirable as regards organization,

equipment, and effort, but totally devoid of romance. This was a business proposition, nothing more.

On our way back a couple of days later we called in to see our friend as we had promised. We climbed up to his corrugated iron shack, but he wasn't there, so we wandered over to the opening and heard him working down below. He took us down through a side tunnel, and we inspected the workings. He was using a pick and shovel in the traditional style, and in the rock he was removing you could see occasional tiny specks of gold. The mine was not more than twenty feet deep, and most of the workings were on the surface; he pulled up his rock by a primitive windlass at the top of the shaft. He showed us the dolley for crushing samples of what he fetched up; he sent the bulk of it to the battery for processing, and a truck called for it every month, as it might do for the washing. He let the children pick over the pile which was waiting to be called for, and each take a little piece in which the gold was visible. They were fascinated. The lure of gold had them fast, and for weeks afterwards they dug for it in our back garden; this was the only life to lead, striking it rich one week, starving another. Still, many years later, they remember their friend with affection and respect.

I can quite see the attraction of gold mining, considering it purely on this sort of individual level. But what a silly business it is when you think of the product as a commodity! Apart from jewellery and some chemical and medical uses, there is nothing you can do with it except lock it up in places like Fort Knox, sterile and valueless except as a concept, an abstraction. Why should reasonable men put such immense effort into digging up rock in so many parts of the world, converting it to a soft yellow metal, and sending it under guard at great expense to another country overseas, where it is at once buried again underground? Surely our descendants will think us mad? I am no economist, and such questions bother me; I cannot trace the necessary connection in my mind between the occasional frantic gold buying on the world's stock exchanges and the grey tellurite powder clanking along in its trucks at Kalgoorlie, or for that matter, anywhere else in the world where the accidents of geology have hidden it for men to find.

I have had an outsider's view of gold mining in several places, and have always been interested in the mechanics of winning gold, though mystified by its rationale. My first gold mine was a deserted one near Mount Bartle Frere in Queensland. We rode out to it in a jeep, and swam in the river to the shrill insect noises of the bush; we tried to pan some specks of what we swore was gold but which we knew in our hearts was nothing but sand. We had a wonderful time, and dreamed of riches.

In 1953 I visited the other Boulder, in Colorado, and drove up into the Rockies to Central City, where the opera house still functioned on great occasions, as a reminder of the wild days of the past, when the rush was on, and millions were made and lost. A plaque in one of the saloons gave alarming statistics of the numbers of men and women shot within its walls during its period of operation – victims of the violent emotions which have always surrounded the idea of gold. All around the ghost towns of the Rockies there were tunnels in the mountain side and holes in the ground; some of them were made into tourist attractions, but others were posted with official notices reading: 'Keep Out. United States Atomic Energy Commission.'

There were still fossickers who found it worth while to go out – many of them at weekends only – to pick over the leavings which could be found in the beds of the streams. In other places these pickings had been thought worthy of commercial attention, and a dredge had ploughed its way along the water courses, throwing up great ridges of ugly grey material and destroying the homes of the beavers. My personal picture of American gold is of a solitary man beside a solitary stream among the aspens, with a little sluice arrangement and a pan, swilling round his catch to detect the few precious grains of saleable material.

Much the same sort of thing happened in Otago, where the gold is worked out from the area round Arrowtown which once drew people in the great gold rush to the South Island of New Zealand. Dredges have thrown up their desolate refuse along the river banks, where it lies, unsightly and barren, waiting for the centuries to cover it with vegetation. There are still some New Zealanders who believe that the original lode from which all the gold was derived will eventually be discovered, but they are getting fewer. When the mighty Clutha river was curbed by the dam at Roxburgh, so that the flow was temporarily slackened, the banks were thick with people anxious to see what lay in its normally inaccessible bed.

The glories are indeed departing, but in spite of this it seems that there are still personal fortunes to be made. Only recently a man in Victoria picked up a large nugget lying close to the side of a road, and every month or so you may read in the papers of a fortunate strike in some part of Australia. One can understand why a certain type of man will still leave family and friends and go off wandering in the wilderness. I knew a man like this; he was in my Army unit. He had lied about his age in order to enlist, and I think he was about sixty – a grizzled, tough specimen, who had slept most of his nights in the open since he was a lad. He had never found anything worth having, and had often had a hard time keeping himself in food. Yet he regarded it as the only life worth living, and when Japan collapsed his only ambition was to get out as quickly as possible and go back to his search. He reckoned he would find it yet.

Perhaps he did, for the search for gold is a mystique rather than a normal enterprise, an emotional rather than a material way of life, and the seeking is the finding.

Mermaids

IN the file where I keep my certificates one stands out from the mundane records of birth, marriage, qualifications, and so on. It deals with my first crossing of the Equator, in August of 1943, on my way to Sydney from San Francisco as the only British officer among some 500 American troops.

'Know ye all', says the certificate, 'that on the forty fifth day of Jupiter in the year of Our reign ten thousand and forty three there appeared within Our Royal Domain an American Army transport in latitude 0°0'0'' and longitude 118°0'0'' '. It goes on to state that the Royal Staff of Neptunus Rex, who issued the certificate, found me worthy to be numbered as a Trusty Shellback, and to command that due honour and respect should be shown me whenever I enter his realm. The portrait of Neptunus Rex appears in the top left hand corner, and he has appended his seal. The certificate is countersigned by Davey Jones, as scribe to His Majesty, and attested by the ship's commander, the o/c troops and the o/c armed guard. All this is impressive enough, but what really holds the attention is a plump and shapely mermaid in the other top corner.

Since then I have had but little to do with mermaids. While in Australia, I was sent by the War Office, a technical drawing of a Japanese naval mine surrounded by watery creatures which included an octopus, a lobster, and a mermaid, rather less well favoured than His Majesty's consort. A note of clarification at the bottom said: 'The accompanying fauna are not to scale'.

On my way home to be demobilized I briefly encountered a three dimensional mermaid in the Crescent in Aden, a chimaera rather crudely put together from an assortment of marine inhabitants. Later still I saw the statue of the little mermaid in Copenhagen harbour, a touching testimony to the power of the written word of Hans Anderson. And I have seen a couple of mermaids at the movies.

I crossed the Equator another five times in the realm of Neptunus Rex before I deserted him for the airways, but on none of these occasions did a certificate or a mermaid appear. As for the subsequent crossings by air, Neptune obviously does not claim the airspace above his domain, for no mermaid or even airmaid (I except the stewardesses) has ever appeared there either.

My bag of mermaids is thus a poor one, and I look forward to further and more extended encounters on my next trip under the protection of Neptunus Rex.

Cowardice

ON a psychological scale of bravery, with cowardly at 1 and reckless at 10, my normal score would be 3 or 4, between 'cautious' and 'prudent'. But when I go abroad, the score drops at once to 1 or at most 2. I am the last person in any group to attempt to lodge a complaint in Serbo-Croat or to perambulate the rim of an active volcano. I refuse to take my car overseas, since I might be required to drive it through Paris, or even Rome, and as a passenger on roads bounded by precipices in Norway or Peru I simply shut my eyes and wait for death.

If sea slugs or fried bees are on the menu I cravenly call for an omelette, and where the cuisine is Indonesian or Thai I scrutinize the pile of material in front of me with great care before helping myself exceedingly sparingly. I take the utmost pains to avoid falling ill, for even at home the spectre of Side Effects leads me to be less than compliant in the taking of prescribed medicines, and who knows what disastrous potions might not be thought appropriate in foreign parts?

In Northern Australia I do not bathe in the sea, unlike the locals, for the presence of sea-going crocodiles, stone fish, blue ringed octopuses, 'stingers' and sea snakes is for me a powerful deterrent to innocent enjoyment. Even on land the snake problem is seldom out of my mind as I walk in the bush, and I envisage scrub typhus and dengue lurking under every piece of foliage.

When at the Grand Canyon I do not seek to stand on overhanging stones, with nothing underneath them for an incalculable number of feet. True, I did once nerve myself to look down a 2000 feet vertical cliff in Madeira, restrained from falling over by a rickety spar clearly suffering from wood fatigue. But such an occasion stands out, like a Dartmoor tor, from a morass of cowardice. On the Milford Track in New Zealand I rejected the opportunity of standing under the world's third highest waterfall, and I did not take the boat trip through the maelstrom at Niagara. At Ayers Rock in central Australia I refused to climb to the top once I had discovered the memorial tablets commemorating the 12 people who had died as a result of so doing. As a youth I stood on the sidelines instead of running in front of the bulls at the encierro at Pamplona. I never tried to surf in Hawaii, to ski in Switzerland, or to climb in the Andes. I often think it might be nice to ascend the bravery scale to at least the word 'enterprising', but I now have little hope of this, and have decided that my genes are just not the type.

Airports

IN the course of a life spent avoiding air travel whenever possible I seem to have accumulated experience of a fair number of airports – 83 by the last count. Some are old acquaintances (I do not say friends), visited many times and perforce familiar.

Others, such as Heathrow, where I was once immobilized for an
entire day by a strike and a bomb scare, come under the heading
of enemies. In this category I also include places like Miami,
infested by religious fanatics pestering me to buy obscure
sectarian tracts or Hindu sacred books.

On the whole I bear the others no particular grudge. From
most of them I have sallied out into the surrounding territory for
a few days or months, but others are represented in my memory
merely by transit lounges of a deadening uniformity, with Duty
Free goods I do not want, 'new' paperbacks which turn out to
be old ones masquerading under a new cover, ghastly coffee,
and incomprehensible public address announcements which
have to be listened to with unnatural attention since it is just
possible that their content may affect my own future.

In some cases I have been quite glad not to be allowed out: I
had no real desire to explore Madras at 2 a.m., and I felt that
Beirut was best left unexplored in broad daylight. But in others
bad planning or adverse circumstances deprived me of what
would have been a welcome opportunity. At Easter Island, for
instance, my entire stopover of one hour was spent going
through Chilean immigration; not a statue was in sight except
for a dwarf replica in a corner outside. At Antananarivo I would
have liked to mount an expedition to watch the waving tails of
the lemurs, and in Moroni in the Comoros I would have enjoyed
looking round for a day or two, even though I find coelacanths
deadly dull creatures.

I have seen a few airports grow up from a hut with a weighing
machine inside to giant international palaces, and others de-
generate into virtual disuse. Some, like Suva, have retained a
reputation for an element of risk, and others, such as Faaa in
Tahiti or Paraburdoo in Western Australia, commend themselves to my affection on account of their names. I have fond
memories of Adelaide, where, owing to a fault in the public
address system, the last call for my flight caught me, literally,
with my trousers down. By the time I ran out on to the tarmac
everybody had embarked, the engines were revving up and the
boarding gangway had been removed. The gangway was
replaced and I was pushed aboard; both passengers and crew
gave me a cheer.

But perhaps my favourite airport is Salt Lake City, which
received me all in one piece and revived me when I arrived more

dead than alive after a flight from Chicago through a giant thunderstorm. Or there is the palatial building at Singapore, where I have twice been off-loaded into a four-star hotel for the night, and where, as a result, I saw the film 'My Fair Lady' with Chinese subtitles and went to sea in a junk.

On the whole, though, I am happiest meeting people at my home airport, and have no intention of trying to increase my score in the future.